NATIONAL ACADEMIES

Sciences
Engineering
Medicine

NATIONAL
ACADEMIES
PRESS
Washington, DC

Addressing Treatment Resistance in the Development of Cancer Immune Modulator Therapeutics

Erin Balogh, Jennifer Zhu, Anne Frances Johnson, and Sharyl Nass, *Rapporteurs*

National Cancer Policy Forum

Board on Health Care Services

Forum on Drug Discovery, Development, and Translation

Board on Health Sciences Policy

Health and Medicine Division

T0286771

Proceedings of a Workshop

THE NATIONAL ACADEMIES PRESS 500 Fifth Street, NW Washington, DC 20001

This activity was supported by Contract No. 75D30121D11240 (Task Order Nos. 75D30121F00002 and 75D30123F00024) with the Centers for Disease Control and Prevention; Contract No. HHSN263201800029I (Task Order Nos. HHSN26300007, HHSN26300008, 75N98023F00019, and 75N98023F00020) with the National Institutes of Health (National Cancer Institute, National Institute of Allergy and Infectious Diseases, National Institute of Mental Health, National Institute of Neurological Disorders and Stroke, and Office of Science Policy); and Grant No. 1R13FD007302-01 with the U.S. Food and Drug Administration. This activity was also supported by the American Association for Cancer Research; American Cancer Society; American College of Radiology; American Society of Clinical Oncology; Amgen Inc.; Association of American Cancer Institutes; Association of American Medical Colleges; Association of Community Cancer Centers; AstraZeneca; Biogen; Bristol Myers Squibb; Burroughs Wellcome Fund; Cancer Support Community; Critical Path Institute; Eli Lilly & Co.; FasterCures, Milken Institute; Flatiron Health; Foundation for the National Institutes of Health; Friends of Cancer Research; Johnson & Johnson; Medable, Inc.; Merck; National Comprehensive Cancer Network; National Patient Advocate Foundation; *New England Journal of Medicine*; Novartis Oncology; Oncology Nursing Society; Partners in Health; Pfizer Inc; Sanofi; and Society for Immunotherapy of Cancer. Any opinions, findings, conclusions, or recommendations expressed in this publication do not necessarily reflect the views of any organization or agency that provided support for the project.

International Standard Book Number-13: 978-0-309-71626-0
International Standard Book Number-10: 0-309-71626-8
Digital Object Identifier: https://doi.org/10.17226/27517

This publication is available from the National Academies Press, 500 Fifth Street, NW, Keck 360, Washington, DC 20001; (800) 624-6242 or (202) 334-3313; http://www.nap.edu.

Suggested citation: National Academies of Sciences, Engineering, and Medicine. 2024. *Addressing treatment resistance in the development of cancer immune modulator therapeutics: Proceedings of a workshop.* Washington, DC: The National Academies Press. https://doi.org/10.17226/27517.

The **National Academy of Sciences** was established in 1863 by an Act of Congress, signed by President Lincoln, as a private, nongovernmental institution to advise the nation on issues related to science and technology. Members are elected by their peers for outstanding contributions to research. Dr. Marcia McNutt is president.

The **National Academy of Engineering** was established in 1964 under the charter of the National Academy of Sciences to bring the practices of engineering to advising the nation. Members are elected by their peers for extraordinary contributions to engineering. Dr. John L. Anderson is president.

The **National Academy of Medicine** (formerly the Institute of Medicine) was established in 1970 under the charter of the National Academy of Sciences to advise the nation on medical and health issues. Members are elected by their peers for distinguished contributions to medicine and health. Dr. Victor J. Dzau is president.

The three Academies work together as the **National Academies of Sciences, Engineering, and Medicine** to provide independent, objective analysis and advice to the nation and conduct other activities to solve complex problems and inform public policy decisions. The National Academies also encourage education and research, recognize outstanding contributions to knowledge, and increase public understanding in matters of science, engineering, and medicine.

Learn more about the National Academies of Sciences, Engineering, and Medicine at **www.nationalacademies.org**.

PLANNING COMMITTEE[1]

SAMIR N. KHLEIF (*Co-Chair*), Georgetown University
GEORGE J. WEINER (*Co-Chair*), University of Iowa
GIDEON BLUMENTHAL, Merck
CHRIS BOSHOFF, Pfizer Inc.
TOM CURRAN, Children's Mercy Kansas City
NANCY E. DAVIDSON, Fred Hutchinson Cancer Center; University of
Washington
JULIE R. GRALOW, American Society of Clinical Oncology
ROY S. HERBST, Yale University
HEDVIG HRICAK, Memorial Sloan Kettering Cancer Center
SCOTT M. LIPPMAN, University of California, San Diego
W. KIMRYN RATHMELL, Vanderbilt University Medical Center
MARC THEORET, Oncology Center of Excellence, U.S. Food and Drug
Administration

Project Staff

ANNA ADLER, Senior Program Assistant (*from September 2023*)
FRANCIS AMANKWAH, Program Officer (*through August 2022*)
LORI BENJAMIN BRENIG, Research Associate (*through May 2023*)
TORRIE BROWN, Program Coordinator
CHIDINMA CHUKWURAH, Senior Program Assistant
GRACE McCARTHY, Christine Mirzayan Science and Technology Policy
Graduate Fellow (*March–May 2023*)
EMMA WICKLAND, Research Associate (*from September 2023*)
JULIE WILTSHIRE, Senior Finance Business Partner
JENNIFER ZHU, Associate Program Officer (*from January 2023*)
CAROLYN SHORE, Director, Forum on Drug Discovery, Development,
and Translation
ERIN BALOGH, Co-Director, National Cancer Policy Forum
SHARYL NASS, Co-Director, National Cancer Policy Forum; Senior
Director, Board on Health Care Services

---

[1] The National Academies of Sciences, Engineering, and Medicine's planning committees are solely responsible for organizing the workshop, identifying topics, and choosing speakers. The responsibility for the published Proceedings of a Workshop rests with the workshop rapporteurs and the institution.

NATIONAL CANCER POLICY FORUM[1]

ROBERT A. WINN (*Chair*), Virginia Commonwealth University
PETER C. ADAMSON, Sanofi
JUSTIN E. BEKELMAN, University of Pennsylvania
SMITA BHATIA, The University of Alabama at Birmingham
GIDEON BLUMENTHAL, Merck
CHRIS BOSHOFF, Pfizer Inc.
OTIS W. BRAWLEY, Johns Hopkins University
HILLARY CAVANAGH, Centers for Medicare & Medicaid Services
CHRISTINA CHAPMAN, Baylor College of Medicine; Michael E.
    DeBakey VA Medical Center
GWEN DARIEN, National Patient Advocate Foundation
CRYSTAL DENLINGER, National Comprehensive Cancer Network
JAMES H. DOROSHOW, National Cancer Institute
S. GAIL ECKHARDT, Baylor College of Medicine
CHRISTOPHER R. FRIESE, University of Michigan
STANTON L. GERSON, Case Western Reserve University
SCARLETT LIN GOMEZ, University of California, San Francisco
JULIE R. GRALOW, American Society of Clinical Oncology
ROY S. HERBST, Yale University; American Association for Cancer
    Research
HEDVIG HRICAK, Memorial Sloan Kettering Cancer Center
CHANITA HUGHES-HALBERT, University of Southern California
ROY A. JENSEN, University of Kansas; Association of American Cancer
    Institutes
RANDY A. JONES, University of Virginia
BETH Y. KARLAN, University of California, Los Angeles
SAMIR N. KHLEIF, Georgetown University; Society for Immunotherapy
    of Cancer
SCOTT M. LIPPMAN, University of California, San Diego
ELENA MARTINEZ, University of California, San Diego
LARISSA NEKHLYUDOV, Brigham and Women's Hospital; Dana-
    Farber Cancer Institute; Harvard Medical School

---

[1] The National Academies of Sciences, Engineering, and Medicine's forums and roundtables do not issue, review, or approve individual documents. The responsibility for the published Proceedings of a Workshop rests with the workshop rapporteurs and the institution.

RANDALL A. OYER, University of Pennsylvania; Penn Medicine
    Lancaster General Health; Association of Community Cancer Centers
CLEO A. RYALS, Flatiron Health
RICHARD L. SCHILSKY, ASCO TAPUR Study; University of Chicago
JULIE SCHNEIDER, Oncology Center of Excellence, U.S. Food and
    Drug Administration
SUSAN M. SCHNEIDER, Duke University
LAWRENCE N. SHULMAN, University of Pennsylvania
HEIDI SMITH, Novartis Pharmaceuticals
KATRINA TRIVERS, Centers for Disease Control and Prevention
ROBIN YABROFF, American Cancer Society

Forum Staff

ANNA ADLER, Senior Program Assistant
TORRIE BROWN, Program Coordinator
CHIDINMA CHUKWURAH, Senior Program Assistant
EMMA WICKLAND, Research Associate
JULIE WILTSHIRE, Senior Finance Business Partner
JENNIFER ZHU, Associate Program Officer
ERIN BALOGH, Co-Director, National Cancer Policy Forum
SHARYL NASS, Co-Director, National Cancer Policy Forum;
    Senior Director, Board on Health Care Services

FORUM ON DRUG DISCOVERY, DEVELOPMENT, AND TRANSLATION[1]

GREGORY SIMON (*Co-Chair*), Kaiser Permanente Washington Health Research Institute; University of Washington

ANN TAYLOR (*Co-Chair*), Retired

BARBARA E. BIERER, Harvard Medical School; Brigham and Women's Hospital

LINDA BRADY, National Institute of Mental Health, NIH

JOHN BUSE, University of North Carolina, Chapel Hill School of Medicine

LUTHER T. CLARK, Merck

BARRY S. COLLER, The Rockefeller University

TAMMY R.L. COLLINS, Burroughs Wellcome Fund

TOM CURRAN, Children's Mercy, Kansas City

RICHARD DAVEY, National Institute of Allergy and Infectious Diseases, NIH

KATHERINE DAWSON, Biogen

JAMES H. DOROSHOW, National Cancer Institute, NIH

JEFFREY M. DRAZEN, *New England Journal of Medicine*

STEVEN K. GALSON, Retired

CARLOS O. GARNER, Eli Lilly & Company

SALLY L. HODDER, West Virginia University

TESHEIA JOHNSON, Yale School of Medicine

LYRIC JORGENSON, Office of Science Policy, NIH

ESTHER KROFAH, FasterCures, Milken Institute

LISA M. LaVANGE, University of North Carolina

ARAN MAREE, Johnson & Johnson

CRISTIAN MASSACESI, AstraZeneca

ROSS McKINNEY JR., Association of American Medical Colleges

JOSEPH P. MENETSKI, Foundation for the National Institutes of Health

ANAEZE C. OFFODILE II, University of Texas MD Anderson Cancer Center

SALLY OKUN, Clinical Trials Transformation Initiative

---

[1] The National Academies of Sciences, Engineering, and Medicine's forums and roundtables do not issue, review, or approve individual documents. The responsibility for the published Proceedings of a Workshop rests with the workshop rapporteurs and the institution.

ARTI RAI, Duke University School of Law

KLAUS ROMERO, Critical Path Institute

JONI RUTTER, National Center for Advancing Translational Sciences, NIH

SUSAN SCHAEFFER, The Patients' Academy for Research Advocacy

ANANTHA SHEKHAR, University of Pittsburgh School of Medicine

ELLEN V. SIGAL, Friends of Cancer Research

MARK TAISEY, Amgen Inc.

AMIR TAMIZ, National Institute of Neurological Disorders and Stroke, NIH

PAMELA TENAERTS, Medable Inc.

MAJID VAKILYNEJAD, Takeda

JONATHAN WATANABE, University of California Irvine School of Pharmacy and Pharmaceutical Sciences

ALASTAIR WOOD, Vanderbilt University

CRIS WOOLSTON, Sanofi

JOSEPH C. WU, Stanford University School of Medicine

Forum Staff

CAROLYN SHORE, Forum Director

KYLE CAVAGNINI, Associate Program Officer

BRITTANY HSIAO, Associate Program Officer (*as of September 2023*)

MAYA THIRKILL, Associate Program Officer (*until April 2023*)

NOAH ONTJES, Research Associate

MELVIN JOPPY, Senior Program Assistant

CLARE STROUD, Senior Director, Board on Health Sciences Policy

Reviewers

This Proceedings of a Workshop was reviewed in draft form by individuals chosen for their diverse perspectives and technical expertise. The purpose of this independent review is to provide candid and critical comments that will assist the National Academies of Sciences, Engineering, and Medicine in making each published proceedings as sound as possible and to ensure that it meets the institutional standards for quality, objectivity, evidence, and responsiveness to the charge. The review comments and draft manuscript remain confidential to protect the integrity of the process.

We thank the following individuals for their review of this proceedings:

NICOLE J. GORMLEY, U.S. Food and Drug Administration
ANTONI RIBAS, University of California, Los Angeles
ALEXANDRA SNYDER, Generate Biomedicines
SUZANNE L. TOPALIAN, Johns Hopkins University

Although the reviewers listed above provided many constructive comments and suggestions, they were not asked to endorse the content of the proceedings nor did they see the final draft before its release. The review of this proceedings was overseen by **DANIEL R. MASYS,** University of Washington. He was responsible for making certain that an independent examination of this proceedings was carried out in accordance with standards of the National Academies and that all review comments were carefully considered. Responsibility for the final content rests entirely with the rapporteurs and the National Academies.

Acknowledgments

The National Cancer Policy Forum is grateful for the support of our many annual sponsors. Federal sponsors include the Centers for Disease Control and Prevention and the National Cancer Institute/National Institutes of Health. Non-federal sponsors include the American Association for Cancer Research, American Cancer Society, American College of Radiology, American Society of Clinical Oncology, Association of American Cancer Institutes, Association of Community Cancer Centers, Bristol Myers Squibb, Cancer Support Community, Flatiron Health, Merck & Co., Inc., National Comprehensive Cancer Network, National Patient Advocate Foundation, Novartis Oncology, Oncology Nursing Society, Partners in Health, Pfizer Inc., Sanofi, and Society for Immunotherapy of Cancer.

The Forum on Drug Discovery, Development, and Translation is also appreciative of the support from our many annual sponsors. Federal sponsors include the National Institutes of Health (National Cancer Institute, National Institute on Allergy and Infectious Diseases, National Institute of Mental Health, National Institute of Neurological Disorders and Stroke, and Office of Science Policy) and the U.S. Food and Drug Administration. Non-federal sponsors include Amgen Inc.; Association of American Medical Colleges; AstraZeneca; Biogen; Burroughs Wellcome Fund; Critical Path Institute; Eli Lilly & Co.; FasterCures, Milken Institute; Foundation for the National Institutes of Health; Friends of Cancer Research; Johnson & Johnson; Medable Inc.; Merck; *New England Journal of Medicine*; and Sanofi.

The Forums wish to express their gratitude to the expert speakers whose presentations and discussions helped inform efforts to counter resistance and advance meaningful progress in the development of immune modulator therapies for cancer treatment. The Forums also wish to thank the members of the planning committee for their work in developing an excellent workshop agenda.

Contents

Boxes and Figures

BOXES

FIGURES

Acronyms and Abbreviations

AhR	aryl hydrocarbon receptor
AI	artificial intelligence
CAR T	chimeric antigen receptor T cell
CD	cluster of differentiation
COE	contribution of effect
COVID-19	coronavirus disease of 2019
ctDNA	circulating tumor DNA
CTLA-4	cytotoxic T-lymphocyte-associated protein 4
dMMR	deficient mismatch repair
EHR	electronic health record
FDA	U.S. Food and Drug Administration
FNIH	Foundation for the National Institutes of Health
GITR	glucocorticoid-induced tumor-necrosis-factor-related gene
ICI	immune checkpoint inhibitor
IDO1	indoleamine 2,3-dioxygenase-1
irAE	immune-related adverse event
JAK	Janus kinase

LAG-3   lymphocyte activation gene-3
LungMAP   Lung Cancer Master Protocol

mCODE   Minimal Common Oncology Data Elements
ML   machine learning
MRD   minimal residual disease
MRI   magnetic resonance imaging
MSI-H   microsatellite instability-high

NCI   National Cancer Institute
NLP   natural language processing

ORIEN   Oncology Research Information Exchange Network

pCR   pathological complete response
PD-1   programmed cell death receptor 1
PD-L1   programmed cell death ligand 1
PET   positron emission tomography

RECIST   Response Evaluation Criteria in Solid Tumors
RNA   ribonucleic acid

SCNA   somatic copy number alteration

TCR   T-cell receptor
TMB-H   tumor mutational burden-high

Proceedings of a Workshop

WORKSHOP OVERVIEW[1]

Immune modulators are a type of immunotherapy that enhances the immune system response to cancer (NCI, 2023). The advent of immune modulator therapeutics has been heralded as a new era in cancer care, yet these approaches still fall short of expectations in some ways, said Samir Khleif, biomedical scholar, professor of oncology, and director of the Center of Immunology and Immunotherapy at Georgetown University. For certain types of cancer, these therapeutics may represent the best and sometimes only treatment option, but uneven response rates, disease resistance, and serious side effects have limited the benefit for many patients (Seliger and Massa, 2021). George Weiner, professor of internal medicine, pharmaceutical science, and experimental therapeutics at the University of Iowa, highlighted the enormous growth in the use of immunotherapies for cancer treatment but said that resistance to treatment poses a serious threat to future advances in the field.

To discuss current challenges related to resistance to immunotherapies and policy opportunities to overcome them, the National Academies of Sciences, Engineering, and Medicine held a workshop, Addressing Treatment Resistance

---

[1] This workshop was organized by an independent planning committee whose role was limited to identification of topics and speakers. This Proceedings of a Workshop was prepared by the rapporteurs as a factual summary of the presentations and discussions that took place at the workshop. Statements, recommendations, and opinions expressed are those of individual presenters and participants and are not endorsed or verified by the National Academies of Sciences, Engineering, and Medicine, and they should not be construed as reflecting any group consensus.

1

in the Development of Cancer Immune Modulator Therapeutics, convened by the National Cancer Policy Forum in collaboration with the Forum on Drug Discovery, Development, and Translation on November 14 and 15, 2022. This workshop builds on the National Cancer Policy Forum's prior work, including the workshops Policy Issues in the Clinical Development and Use of Immunotherapy for Cancer Treatment (NASEM, 2016) and Advancing Progress in the Development of Combination Cancer Therapies with Immune Checkpoint Inhibitors (NASEM, 2019).

This Proceedings of a Workshop summarizes the issues discussed. Many speakers provided observations on immunotherapy resistance and suggestions on the opportunities to overcome key policy, practice, and research challenges to advance research and implementation—highlighted in Boxes 1 and 2, respectively, and discussed throughout the proceedings. Appendixes A and B include the Statement of Task and agenda, respectively. Video recordings and speaker presentations are available online.[2]

---

[2] See https://www.nationalacademies.org/event/11-14-2022/addressing-resistance-in-the-development-of-cancer-immune-modulator-therapeutics-a-workshop (accessed March 30, 2023).

BOX 1
Observations Made by Individual Workshop Participants on the Development of Immune Modulator Therapeutics

- Proof of mechanisms for treatment resistance remains a major challenge for immunotherapy development and understanding resistance. (Healy, Khleif, Tawbi, Theoret)
- A lack of consistent definitions for resistance and response hampers the ability to compare across studies and inform clinical trial design. (Luke, Rathmell, Tawbi, Theoret)
- More single-agent therapies, more pathways to early- and late-stage trials, and more pathways to efficient creation of combination treatments are needed. (Curran, Janik, Khleif, Topalian)
- A more holistic understanding of a healthy immune system, tumor response, and tumor resistance is needed to improve immunotherapy development. (Boshoff, Davidson, Gralow, Herbst, Mayerhoefer, Rathmell, Tawbi)
- Evidence of biological activity in single agents may be more important than clinical response in prioritizing combination therapy development. (Khleif, Sharon, Topalian, Weiner)

BOX 1 Continued

- Dosing and sequencing of therapies have important implications for the tumor microenvironment, response, and resistance. (Blumenthal, Khleif, Snyder, Theoret, Weiner)
- The biology of the immune system is not a simple target but a complex system with multiple inhibition mechanisms; targets that require inhibition of multiple actions will likely require combination treatments rather than single agents. (Pe'er, Tawbi)
- More effective collaboration, communication, and data sharing are needed among all parties involved in immunotherapy drug development. (Boshoff, Davidson, Gralow, Herbst, Hricak, Lippman, Rathmell, Theoret)
- Negative results from immunotherapy clinical trials can have ripple effects across the entire field of immunotherapy development. (Herbst, Hricak, Snyder, Wolchok)
- Important lessons can be drawn from clinical trials with negative results. (Blumenthal, Curran, Fayyad, Grupp, Herbst, Khleif, Luke, Sharon, Snyder, Theoret, Weiner)

NOTE: This list is the rapporteurs' summary of points made by the individual speakers identified, and the statements have not been endorsed or verified by the National Academies of Sciences, Engineering, and Medicine. The points are not intended to reflect a consensus among workshop participants.

BOX 2
Suggestions from Individual Workshop Participants to Address Treatment Resistance and Improve the Development of Immune Modulator Therapeutics

Prioritizing research to understand and characterize resistance
- Invest in preclinical models to characterize new agents and their mechanisms of action, response, and resistance. (Curran, Healy, Janik, Khleif, Snyder, Tawbi, Topalian)
- Invest in research that characterizes the tumor microenvironment. (Khleif, Weiner)
- Leverage systems-level biology approaches to facilitate immunotherapy research and development. (Curran, Khleif, Pe'er)
- Prioritize research to develop and validate biomarkers and surrogate endpoints. (Boshoff, Gormley, Healy, Herbst, Hricak, Janik, Lippman, Rathmell, Sharon, Snyder, Theoret)

continued

BOX 2 Continued

- Develop companion diagnostic assays for clinical decision making. (Bross, Davoli, Philip)

Designing and conducting clinical trials to improve immunotherapy development
- Improve clinical trial design by incorporating validated biomarkers and assessing outcomes that are appropriate for immunotherapy single agents and combinations. (Blumenthal, Gralow, Herbst, Hricak, Khleif, Rathmell, Theoret, Weiner)
- When feasible, conduct randomized rather than single-arm trials, including randomization of dosing in early-phase clinical trials. (Luke, Snyder, Theoret)
- Work with the U.S. Food and Drug Administration to develop and select clinical trial designs that are appropriate for single-agent and combination immunotherapies. (Khleif)

Encouraging collaboration, data sharing, and multidisciplinary research
- Utilize public–private partnerships to share resources and improve representation of diverse patient populations in clinical trials. (Herbst)
- Share results from negative trials, and use them as learning opportunities. (Blumenthal, Fayyad, Khleif, Snyder)
- Improve and standardize systems for reporting adverse events to enable better use of real-world clinical and patient-reported data. (Brant, Weiner, Yerram)
- Improve data sharing, develop and adopt data standards, and facilitate the use of advanced computational tools. (Boshoff, Curran, Davidson, Gralow, Khleif, Pe'er, Rathmell, Tarhini, Yerram)
- Foster a multidisciplinary workforce of clinical investigators, including expertise in data science. (Davidson, Fayyad, Khleif, Rathmell)

NOTE: This list is the rapporteurs' summary of points made by the individual speakers identified, and the statements have not been endorsed or verified by the National Academies of Sciences, Engineering, and Medicine. The points are not intended to reflect a consensus among workshop participants.

SCIENTIFIC INNOVATIONS TO ADVANCE CANCER CARE

Elizabeth Jaffee, chair of the President's Cancer Panel and deputy director of the Johns Hopkins Sidney Kimmel Comprehensive Cancer Center, underscored the urgent need to develop better cancer therapeutics. Despite numerous scientific breakthroughs and substantial government investment, cancer remains a leading cause of death around the globe: "We are at a pivotal time in cancer research and cancer care," said Jaffee. "Reducing the cancer burden will improve the quality of life for so many, leading to enhanced measures of world economic success."

History of Immunotherapy Development

Jaffee reviewed the development timeline of immune modulator therapeutics, noting that it took approximately 10 years to determine the function of immune checkpoints—a group of inhibitory and stimulatory pathways that influence immune cell activity—and another 15 years to achieve the first approval in 2011 by the U.S. Food and Drug Administration (FDA) of an immune checkpoint inhibitor (ICI): anti-cytotoxic T-lymphocyte-associated protein 4 (CTLA-4), ipilimumab.[3] In the following decade, FDA approved several ICIs in two different categories (antibodies that target programmed cell death receptor 1 [PD-1] and its ligand [PD-L1]).[4] Jaffee noted that the trajectory of these medical advancements was augmented by technological innovations, including sequencing the human genome and the development of next-generation sequencing, multi-omic tests, and technologies to visualize the cellular heterogeneity and spatial architecture of the tumor microenvironment.

Despite major achievements over the past several decades, Jaffee said that advancement in the field has plateaued in recent years. To advance progress, she said there is a need to facilitate rapid development of combination immunotherapies, which requires solving overarching challenges in clinical trial design, data sharing, and patient access to clinical trials. Jaffee emphasized the importance of cross-disciplinary collaboration among government, industry, academia, patient advocacy groups, foundations, and others. "It's time to leverage these unprecedented opportunities into more rapid and improved patient outcomes so that all patients with cancer will benefit," she said.

---

[3] CTLA-4 is a protein receptor on T cells. When bound, it transmits an inhibitory signal that prevents T cells from killing other cells, including cancer cells (Bashyam, 2007). See https://news.bms.com/news/details/2011/FDA-Approves-YERVOY-ipilimumab-for-the-Treatment-of-Patients-with-Newly-Diagnosed-or-Previously-Treated-Unresectable-or-Metastatic-Melanoma-the-Deadliest-Form-of-Skin-Cancer/default.aspx (accessed October 17, 2023).

[4] Anti-PD-1 and anti-PD-L1 therapies are antibodies that block the binding of PD-1 to PD-L1, which blocks T cell suppression. This boosts the immune system's ability to attack cancer cells (Han et al., 2021).

Clinical Trial Challenges and Opportunities

Randomized controlled trials[5] remain the gold standard for assessing medical interventions, but Jaffee said that these trials often pose significant challenges in developing combination immunotherapies. Innovative, adaptive clinical trial designs offer opportunities to overcome some of these challenges and generate rapid data to aid combination development. Jaffee highlighted several priority areas to improve clinical trial design, including integrating novel multidimensional biomarkers to select combination treatments to test and identify which patients are most likely to respond to them; extracting quantitative features from noninvasive imaging; conducting more sensitive and specific clonal tracking of tumor DNA; improving understanding of baseline immune health; increasing the speed of biomarker identification; and focusing more on tools for data and biospecimen sharing and analysis. She suggested that focusing on smaller, more nimble studies can help to rapidly iterate "bench-to-bedside" bidirectional translational research in a way that is both patient centered and science driven (see Figure 1).

Facilitating broader patient access to clinical trials would accelerate research and expand the number of people who could benefit from emerging therapies,

---

[5] Randomized controlled trials measure the effectiveness of a treatment within a population. The experimental group is randomly assigned to receive treatment, and the control group does not. This process helps to reduce bias (Hariton and Locascio, 2018).

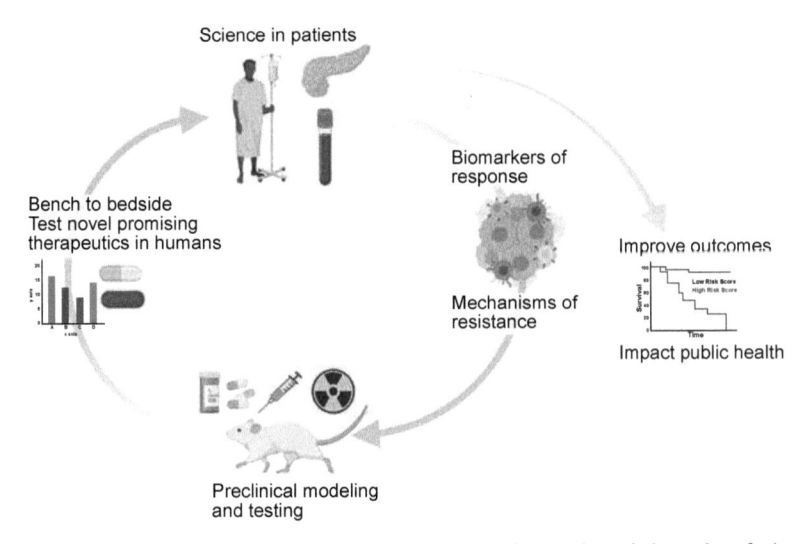

FIGURE 1 "Bench-to-bedside" bidirectional translational research can help to identify the optimal combinations and drive progress in cancer therapy development.
SOURCE: Jaffee presentation, November 14, 2022.

said Jaffee. She suggested using digital technologies that would enable patients to register so that they can be rapidly identified and notified when a relevant trial becomes available. She added that smaller and more targeted trials offered across multiple clinical sites could also improve patient access. Technological innovations, such as wearable digital health tools, and omics-generated data could also be harnessed to improve clinical trial design and aid in patient symptom management.

Data Sharing

To make informed decisions about future research directions, Jaffee said that it is important to overcome challenges to data sharing and integration. Existing datasets are rich with information that could be mined with artificial intelligence (AI) or machine learning (ML) tools to rapidly identify subpopulations of patients who respond to cancer therapies, pathways of resistance to treatment, and promising drug combinations. Jaffee said that accelerating clinical trial data sharing would benefit all parties, reduce waste, boost investment returns, and improve patient outcomes (Spreafico et al., 2021). In addition, Jaffee called for engaging more experts in data science to apply new technologies and methodological approaches to interpret these rich data to facilitate drug development (Davis-Marcisak et al., 2021; Stahlberg et al., 2022).

Jaffee identified several opportunities to facilitate data sharing and accelerate therapy development. She said that government, academia, and industry could collaborate to streamline FDA regulations and reduce drug development costs; create better incentives for companies that achieve first approval for new classes of drugs and biosimilars; address research and data sharing challenges associated with the Privacy Rule;[6] reduce time to publication; create a national or global open-source clinical trial data platform; and develop new data science platforms, data integration techniques, and AI tools to select immunotherapy drug combinations. She also pointed to a need for improved strategies for patient engagement and streamlined processes for institutional review board approvals of clinical trials. Jaffee said that implementing such changes on a national scale will require a concerted, collaborative approach. "This is only going to get done if we have strong and innovative leaders ... who collaborate," she concluded.

---

[6] The Privacy Rule, promulgated under the Health Insurance Portability and Accountability Act of 1996 (HIPAA), establishes national standards to protect individuals' medical records and other individually identifiable health information (collectively defined as "protected health information") and applies to health plans, health care clearinghouses, and those health care providers that conduct certain health care transactions electronically. See https://www.hhs.gov/hipaa/for-professionals/privacy/index.html (accessed December 4, 2023).

CRITERIA TO MOVE SINGLE AGENTS INTO CLINICAL TRIALS

Many speakers reviewed current immune modulator therapies and the challenges with resistance to immunotherapy and outlined criteria to move single immunotherapy agents into clinical trials.

Anti-PD-1 Therapies

Suzanne Topalian, director of the Johns Hopkins Melanoma and Skin Cancer Program, Bloomberg-Kimmel Professor of Cancer Immunotherapy, and professor of surgery and oncology at Johns Hopkins University School of Medicine, discussed anti-PD-1 therapies. "People have often referred to immune checkpoint blockade[7] as a revolution or a breakthrough, but in fact, it was really an evolution," she said. Once researchers gained an understanding of how the PD-1 pathway works, they were able to leverage that knowledge to develop mechanistic biomarkers and FDA-approved anti-PD-1 therapies (Larkin et al., 2015; Topalian et al., 2016).

Anti-PD-1 drugs have been successful in treating advanced cancers that resist standard treatments (Lipson et al., 2013). The PD-1 pathway is active in many tumor types, and unlike ligands for CTLA-4, which are expressed everywhere in the body on antigen-presenting cells, PD-L1 (the major ligand for PD-1) is selectively expressed in cancers and at sites of inflammation—an attribute of many cancers. Thus, anti-PD-1 drugs have fewer side effects compared to anti-CTLA-4 drugs, which induce a more global response (Dong et al., 2002). Topalian said that anti-PD-1 drugs are used to treat at least 22 different cancer types (Chang et al., 2021), but additional research could lead to expanded use in other types of cancer.

Weiner asked if anti-PD-1 drugs were interchangeable. Topalian replied that the anti-PD-1 drugs nivolumab, pembrolizumab, and cemiplimab have very similar mechanisms of action, safety profiles, and efficacy. Researchers are considering trials to compare them directly to anti-PD-L1 agents, but such information is currently unavailable.

Anti-Lymphocyte Activation Gene-3 (LAG-3) Antibodies

To evaluate the contributions of the different components in combination therapies and compare single-agent and combination approaches, it is important

---

[7] Immune checkpoints are inhibitory receptor:ligands in the PD-1 pathway that ensure that the immune system does not become overactive. Inhibiting the immune checkpoint blockade results in greater T cell activity to kill cancerous cells (Postow et al., 2015).

"to be mechanism driven—[to] truly understand what our drugs are doing," said Hussein Tawbi, professor of medical oncology and investigational cancer therapeutics, director of melanoma clinical research and early drug development, and codirector of the Brain Metastasis Clinic at the University of Texas MD Anderson Cancer Center.

The LAG-3 protein is an immune checkpoint receptor protein that down-regulates immune response when activated, which can be due to the chronic antigen stimulation of cancer (Huo et al., 2022; Ruffo et al., 2019). Tawbi said that inhibiting LAG-3 is a promising target for combination therapies and potential single-agent therapies. One anti-LAG-3 agent, relatlimab, was granted FDA approval to be used in combination with the anti-PD-1 agent nivolumab for metastatic melanoma after research showed its effectiveness in the combination but not alone (Woo et al., 2012).[8] Other recent research has focused on gaining a better mechanistic understanding to further develop anti-LAG-3 agents for cancer treatment, including in the neoadjuvant[9] setting (Amaria et al., 2022; Andrews et al., 2022; Burnell et al., 2021; Wang et al., 2019). Tawbi said that the broader clinical use of relatlimab will enable researchers to discover more about its mechanisms and potential for use in other combination strategies (Tawbi et al., 2022).

Agonist T Cell Antibodies

Unlike anti-PD-1 and anti-CTLA-4 agents, developing agonist T cell antibodies[10] "has proven to be much more difficult," said John Janik, vice president of clinical research at Cullinan Oncology. Several clinical trials have found that they were either ineffective, alone and in combination, or associated with significant toxicity (Propper and Balkwill, 2022). Janik said that another challenge was that lower doses of agonist T cell antibodies were associated with higher T cell activity, but higher doses were associated with lower T cell activity (Muik et al., 2022). In clinical trials, the agonist T cell antibody (an anti-OX40 antibody) showed no evidence of antitumor effect, although combining it with other immunotherapy agents achieved a better response (Davis et al., 2022; Linch et al., 2015). Moreover, Janik said that PD-1 blockade timing appears to be critical for effective combination therapy (Messenheimer et al., 2017; Shrimali et al., 2017) and that the experiences with agonist

---

[8] See https://www.cancer.gov/news-events/cancer-currents-blog/2022/fda-opdualag-melanoma-lag-3 (accessed March 22, 2023).

[9] A neoadjuvant is an initial treatment to shrink a tumor prior to the main treatment, usually surgery. See https://www.cancer.gov/publications/dictionaries/cancer-terms/def/neoadjuvant-therapy (accessed March 27, 2023).

[10] Agonist T cell antibodies provide stimulatory signaling required for T cells to enhance their response to cancer cells (Choi et al., 2020).

T cell antibodies point to a need for new research approaches, such as smaller studies to evaluate initial potential before launching expensive, large-scale clinical trials.

Chimeric Antigen Receptor T Cell (CAR T) Resistance

Stephan Grupp, director of the cancer immunotherapy program at Children's Hospital of Philadelphia, discussed lessons from the development of a different type of immunotherapy called T-cell transfer therapy, such as CAR T therapy.[11] CAR T-cell therapy involves engineering a patient's T cells in the laboratory to specifically target and kill their tumors. This approach has been challenging in solid tumors but much more successful in blood cancers, especially when applied to naive and early memory T cells,[12] which have enormous proliferation capacity and long-term persistence potential, said Grupp (Cieri et al., 2013; Gattinoni et al., 2011; Marofi et al., 2021). Grupp's team found that patients with leukemia who had more long-term persistence had more of these naive and early memory T cells and that the presence of chronic interferon signaling lowered the likelihood of long-term CAR T-cell persistence (Chen et al., 2021). Although interferon signaling modulates important immune functions, chronic signaling causes exhausted T cells that ultimately become dysfunctional (Luke et al., 2019; Wherry, 2011). He said that these studies suggest that T cell differentiation is an important aspect of CAR T therapy success in blood cancers and may be an important consideration for applying it to solid tumors as well.

Researchers have successfully used CAR T therapy to target cluster of differentiation (CD)19 and CD22 cells to overcome the problem of cancer cell antigen loss,[13] which Grupp said can lead to resistance, although the varying response rates and durability in these studies point to a need for further research (Frey et al., 2021; Spiegel et al., 2021). Grupp added that further research is also needed to extend both CAR T therapy and engineered T-cell receptor (TCR) therapy to solid tumors (D'Angelo et al., 2018; Marofi et al., 2021).

Scott Lippman, distinguished professor and associate vice chancellor for cancer research at University of California San Diego Health, asked about the scale-up potential for CAR T and other cell engineering therapies. Grupp replied

---

[11] See https://www.cancer.gov/about-cancer/treatment/types/immunotherapy/t-cell-transfer-therapy (accessed January 29, 2024).

[12] Naive T cells have not yet differentiated into the different types of possible T cells that have different functions in the immune system. Early memory T cells, sometimes called "stem memory T cells," are considered to be the earliest differentiated memory T cell population (Chu et al., 2020).

[13] Antigen loss is when cancerous cells lose surface characteristics required for immune cell recognition, making it more difficult for the immune system to recognize and kill them (Paul, 2003).

that although cell manufacturing is a very expensive, manually intensive process, the hope is that if an agent is beneficial, drug companies would invest in technologies to scale up production (Abou-El-Enein et al., 2021).

Regulatory Perspective

Peter Bross, chief of the oncology branch at FDA's Center for Biologics Evaluation and Research, described how the Office of Tissues and Advanced Therapies regulates cellular cancer immunotherapies. He said that the majority of investigational new drug applications are for anticancer indications in blood cancers and solid tumors (Lapteva et al., 2020; Levin et al., 2021). Bross said that engineered T cells, such as TCR and CAR T, have been effective single-agent therapies for some cancer types, but, as other speakers noted, the results in solid tumors have not been compelling (Marofi et al., 2021; Weber et al., 2020). Bross said that single-arm studies for patients with relapsed and refractory[14] disease, which can lead to accelerated approval designation, can help to move more such therapies into clinical trials.

In addition, Bross said that using companion diagnostics for specific antigen targets can facilitate single-agent trials. Companion diagnostics are considered medical devices that can be developed under an investigational device exemption to assess biomarker status that may indicate which patients are most likely to benefit from a given therapy.[15] He said that companion diagnostics can maximize benefits and minimize risk by providing information essential to use an agent safely and effectively, adding that it is best to incorporate these early in development.

Opportunities and Challenges to Advance the Development of Single Agents

Many speakers discussed key challenges and research opportunities for single-agent therapies, noting how few single agents have been successful in the clinical setting. "This is where we're failing, because we don't know exactly what they're doing, when to [use] them, and more importantly, how to combine them," Khleif said.

Several speakers stressed the importance of determining an agent's mechanism of action with appropriate preclinical models before starting clinical trials and then

---

[14] "Refractory" describes a disease that does not respond to treatment. See https://www.cancer.gov/publications/dictionaries/cancer-terms/def/refractory (accessed March 23, 2023).

[15] See https://www.fda.gov/medical-devices/in-vitro-diagnostics/companion-diagnostics (accessed November 28, 2023).

confirming the mechanism of action in phase I trials. Tawbi said that cancer immunotherapy is a vast landscape, and before trials start, it is crucial to understand the target, collect mechanism data, and identify the right patient population.

Information about agents' mechanisms of action can help to identify "winning" combinations from the thousands of potential agents. Several speakers said that appropriate preclinical models that can assess sensitivity and resistance will be crucial. Once the mechanism of action is known, a second issue is how to efficiently identify combination treatments, which includes working out the optimal dosage and sequencing. Several speakers suggested that this process may benefit from unconventional clinical trial designs, such as including patients with early-stage diseases.

Dana Pe'er, chair of the Computational and Systems Biology Program and the scientific director of the Gerry Metastasis and Tumor Ecosystems Center at Memorial Sloan Kettering Cancer Center, noted that although discussion often centers on an agent's mechanism of action, immune cells are not a simple target; they are a complex system with multiple inhibition mechanisms. As a result, researchers need more quantitative, combinatorial data to understand their interactions and develop a dynamic model to predict combinations, doses, and timing. Tom Curran, senior vice president, executive director, and chief scientific officer at Children's Mercy Research Institute and professor of cancer biology at the University of Kansas School of Medicine, agreed, saying that a systems biology approach could help move things forward. Tawbi added that targets that require multiple actions to be inhibited will likely require combination treatments rather than single agents.

Tawbi said that another challenge is the lack of a consistent definition for "resistance," in the context of either single or combination agents. He noted the wide variation in patient response, and most studies do not assess the myriad aspects that could affect resistance.

Janik cited the lack of biomarkers as a key challenge. Despite several extensive analyses, his team was often unable to pinpoint a reason for the negative results of the anti-OX40 antibody, likely because the mechanisms of the agent were not clear from the start. Janik added that identifying biomarkers that show whether and how a tumor will respond to an agent or combination would be a big leap forward. Usama Fayyad, executive director of the Institute for Experiential Artificial Intelligence at the Northeastern University Khoury College of Computer Science, suggested learning as much as possible from clinical trials with negative results.

Grupp suggested four key research needs: (1) determine why T cells are not inactivated in solid tumors, (2) find new options for targeting cellular therapies, (3) develop a better understanding of cell trafficking,[16] and (4) identify more

---

[16] "Cell trafficking" refers to the movement of T cells to the tumor site (Slaney et al., 2014).

potential targets for pediatric tumors. Grupp noted that dual antigen targeting may overcome the limitations of CAR T therapy in blood cancers. In addition, opportunities to advance cell manufacturing could have major implications for the field, he said.

SELECTION OF EXPERIMENTAL AGENTS IN COMBINATION THERAPY

Many speakers discussed the challenges and opportunities in developing combination immunotherapies, including criteria and considerations for selecting and assessing combinations.

Understanding the Effects of Combination Immunotherapy

Khleif noted inherent complexities in assessing combination immune therapies and likened the challenge to solving the equation $x + y = ?$, where x and y are different agents, given in different doses and sequences, resulting in different answers with every variation. He added that the target for the combination is not one molecule but the entire tumor microenvironment, and different components of it will react differently to x and y. Sequencing also matters: giving x first may alter the microenvironment, changing the effect of y. The complexity of all these variables makes understanding resistance mechanisms particularly difficult, Khleif said.

However, combination therapy can be a promising strategy to address resistance to anti-PD-1 therapy, Khleif said, adding that studies of combination therapies—even those that fail—can shed light on systems-level impacts and tumor resistance mechanisms.

Clinical Trials for Patients with Anti-PD-1/L1 Refractory Cancers

Jane Healy, scientific associate vice president of oncology early clinical development at Merck, discussed acquired resistance, where patients initially respond to a therapy but then become resistant (Kluger et al., 2020; Sharma et al., 2017). This is a growing problem that may be biologically distinct from primary resistance (when a therapy is wholly ineffective from the start) (Schoenfeld and Hellmann, 2020; Sharma et al., 2017). Unfortunately, Healy said that very little data exist on primary resistant (or "refractory") populations, and consensus guidelines for prognosis and treatment are needed.

Acquired resistance is hard to study, because response criteria in clinical trials frequently evolve to reflect lessons learned from trials of novel therapies. For example, the evolution toward using disease stability versus tumor shrinkage as an endpoint has made it difficult to compare data across trials (Park et al., 2020). In addition, each trial has many variables that may affect resistance, such as timing and dosage, different cancer type or stage, and prior exposures to different treatment regimens. Finally, as other speakers noted, Healy said that the mechanisms of resistance to anti-PD-1 therapies have not been clearly defined (Chen and Mellman, 2013).

Trials assessing combination immunotherapies in populations of individuals with anti-PD-1-resistant cancers are underway and could provide useful data on causes of resistance, toxicity, and relevant biomarkers. To speed up progress, Healy suggested performing molecularly targeted analyses to better understand resistance pathways, sequencing a tumor's exome before and after treatment to identify changes, reaching consensus on criteria and endpoints for clinical trials involving anti-PD-1 and anti-PD-L1 therapies, and clearly defining resistance to those therapies.

Lessons Learned from an Indoleamine
2,3-dioxygenase-1 (IDO1) Inhibitor

Jason Luke, associate professor of medicine and director of the Immunotherapy and Drug Development Center at the University of Pittsburgh Medical Center, discussed lessons learned from testing the unsuccessful combination of the anti-PD-1 drug pembrolizumab and epacadostat, a drug that inhibits IDO1, an immune-suppressing enzyme. Although the initial data were promising, Luke said that the trial was stopped due to lack of efficacy (Hamid et al., 2017; Long et al., 2019), and development of other IDO1 inhibitors was also stopped (Luke et al., 2019; National Library of Medicine, 2021).

Luke said that the data were inadequate to show that epacadostat worked as a single agent (Beatty et al., 2017) and suggested that new measures of drug performance are needed to better understand how therapies are affecting the tumor. For example, he said that peripheral blood assays may not be the best way to measure immuno-oncology effects. He added that the combination may also have had the wrong target—IDO1 plays only a minor role in regulating interferon responses, and the aryl hydrocarbon receptor (AhR) might have made a better target due to its more prominent role (Cheong and Sun, 2018; Labadie et al., 2019). Luke added that several companies are developing AhR inhibitors (McGovern et al., 2022; Murray et al., 2014).

"I don't think we should be rushing forward to just try anything that might modulate the immune system," Luke cautioned. Although IDO1 was clearly immunosuppressive, it was one of a string of drugs that did not show enough therapeutic value (Diab et al., 2022; Idera Pharmaceuticals, 2021). He added that the pharmaceutical industry may be under too much competitive pressure to quickly develop—or drop—a drug. Because drugs have the potential for patient harms, he stressed that rigorous evaluation is needed before launching a clinical trial, including exposure and response relationships, single-agent testing, and translational evidence to support proof of concept.

Intralesional Approaches

Weiner discussed the rationale for intralesional cancer therapy development, in which agents are delivered directly to the tumor (Sakhiya et al., 2021). This route of administration may break immune tolerance by inducing changes in the tumor microenvironment via agents such as viruses, biologics, or nucleic acid therapeutics (Makkouk and Weiner, 2015).

Although these approaches show potential, Weiner said that many unanswered questions remain. Regulatory considerations that are important to address include understanding the mechanisms of action, dosing, pharmacokinetics, pharmacodynamics,[17] injection procedure, safety, toxicity, local and systemic responses, changes over time, and potential for combination therapies. If a drug is designed to have multiple mechanisms, that can make it more effective but also more difficult to determine each mechanism's exact biological effects, Weiner noted.

Another key area for future research is optimizing the administration strategy, including dosage and dose distribution, injection volume, diluent, how often to inject lesions, and whether it is best to inject every lesion, while evaluating each variable for efficacy and potential toxicity and safety issues. Weiner said that another consideration is how to optimally assess patient response; for example, researchers will need to determine whether a response is local or systemic, how to distinguish disease progression from pseudoprogression,[18] and whether combinations improve outcomes. Throughout all of these efforts, Weiner said that it will be essential to effectively track, report, and share data and methods to inform future drug development.

Opportunities to Improve Selection and Development of Combination Therapies

Many speakers discussed opportunities to improve combination therapy selection. Appropriate experimental design is a primary consideration for selection of combination agents, said Gideon Blumenthal, vice president of oncology

---

[17] Pharmacokinetics studies how the body interacts with and affects the drug; pharmacodynamics studies how the drug affects the body (Nebert and Zhang, 2019).

[18] Pseudoprogression is an initial increase in tumor size followed by a decrease in tumor burden, which can lead to prematurely discontinuing an effective treatment (Jia et al., 2019).

global regulatory affairs at Merck, and Marc Theoret, deputy director of the FDA Oncology Center of Excellence. They stressed that it is vital to pursue rigorous preclinical work because all preclinical models have limitations. They also emphasized the need to define immune resistance and patient benefit and said that in interpreting results, it is important to decide whether success is defined by single-agent activity, overall response rate, or a pharmacodynamics endpoint determined from preclinical modeling.

Many speakers noted that randomization in clinical trial design is very important. Theoret said that FDA prefers randomized trials over single-arm trials, but he noted that randomized trials can be adaptive. In addition, randomizing patients to different doses earlier in trials can demonstrate a drug's efficacy more quickly. This suggestion was inspired by FDA's Project Optimus,[19] which aims to optimize dosing in oncology. Several participants suggested that clinicians could use knowledge from this project and other therapeutic areas to inspire improvements.

Several participants also stressed that failures should be treated as learning opportunities. Rather than ignoring failed studies and simply dropping these investigational agents, a number of speakers suggested that developers should be incentivized to hold open discussions about failure mechanisms and also to rescue "failed" drugs for further testing or analysis.

Testing Single and Combination Therapies

Weiner suggested that a single agent may not have to demonstrate an independent clinical response to be selected for a combination therapy. Biological activity—even with no clear therapeutic response—would point to something to pursue, and he suggested designing single-agent studies to monitor all biological activity. Luke agreed, adding that current endpoints may not accurately reflect drug activity or efficacy. For example, he said that the Response Evaluation Criteria in Solid Tumors (RECIST)[20] threshold of 30 percent tumor shrinkage needs to be reevaluated; even 5 percent could show that something significant is happening. Healy also agreed that early-phase clinical trials of monotherapies that do not meet the current RECIST threshold may have value: they can demonstrate activity, aid pharmacodynamic modeling, and help determine dosage. She suggested that researchers should spend more time on this work instead of rushing ahead to later-phase trials.

Luke suggested that researchers be more judicious in the combinations they test and that companies not rush drug development without adequate preclinical

---

[19] For more information regarding Project Optimus, see https://www.fda.gov/about-fda/oncology-center-excellence/project-optimus (accessed March 23, 2023).

[20] See https://recist.eortc.org/ (accessed May 11, 2023).

data. Being first to market has financial incentives, but greenlighting expensive trials without adequate evidence is not good business practice. He also noted that although it sometimes may seem as though a monotherapy had no effect, close examination of the data can prove otherwise. Therefore, Luke said that early trials should incorporate biomarkers and targets so that phase III trials are appropriately designed. Healy agreed, noting that early studies of relatlimab used T cell activity to assess response, and although very few patients responded, the data showed promising biological activity, especially when combined with anti-PD-1 agents.

Khleif expanded on the importance of preclinical work. He said that it is possible to design experiments for assessing increasingly complex drug combinations by starting with appropriate preclinical models that show both responsiveness and nonresponsiveness for each agent. In addition, he said it is important to fully define a drug's developmental path; investigate its mechanisms; understand what contribution another agent would add; assess response; and test agents in resistant models, which can provide more insight compared to responsive models. Khleif suggested that single agents that demonstrate any biologic activity in the tumor microenvironment—not just tumor shrinkage or survival rate—could be moved forward.

Primary Versus Acquired Resistance

Many workshop speakers discussed the current understanding of primary and acquired resistance. Elad Sharon, senior investigator at the National Cancer Institute (NCI) Cancer Therapy Evaluation Program and co-chair of the Cancer Moonshot Adult Immunotherapy Implementation Team, hypothesized that both have similar root causes and that acquired resistance occurs when the more immunotherapy-sensitive tumor cells are killed off, leaving those that are resistant. Healy noted ongoing research in this area, including experiments selecting for certain types of mutations, such as in the Janus kinase (JAK)1/JAK2 proteins that lead to interferon insensitivity, which are found in both acquired and primary resistance and could be used as biomarkers for both. Additional research is needed, including a better understanding of the true prevalence of mutations and biomarkers that can be used to guide therapeutic strategies, to assess whether combination anti-PD-1 therapies would work against both types of resistance, she said. Khleif noted that studying the evolution of the immune system after therapy, in addition to the tumor, could shed light on these questions.

Blumenthal asked whether patients with primary and acquired resistance can be included in the same clinical trials. Khleif replied that separating these patient subpopulations could help to elucidate the different mechanisms of resistance. Healy noted that research on immune monotherapies in individuals with both primary and acquired resistance highlights the value of understanding a therapy's specific target, so it can be tested on the right patient population.

Studying the Tumor Microenvironment

Weiner said that researchers are beginning to measure the tumor microenvironment much more systematically and study the effects of how a therapy changes it. The intralesional approach is promising for this research because it perturbs the tumor with a needle, offering an effective means to remove cells and assess changes, said Weiner.

Khleif agreed, noting that studying changes to the microenvironment could take years but will advance progress in the field. AI and big data analytics could also be leveraged to correlate response and nonresponse and understand the biology. Khleif said that the microenvironment is very complex, but finding biomarkers to measure response would be helpful.

BIOMARKERS AND SURROGATE ENDPOINTS

Many speakers discussed the opportunities and challenges in selecting and validating biomarkers for improving immunotherapy development.

Genetic Biomarkers

Teresa Davoli, assistant professor at the Institute for Systems Genetics at New York University Langone Health, highlighted recent work examining genetic biomarkers for immunotherapy response and resistance. Somatic copy number alterations (SCNAs) represent DNA copy gains and losses and are part of the tumor mutational burden (TMB), which correlates to the immune checkpoint blockade in some cancers. SCNAs could be used as predictive biomarkers of resistance because among patients with immune-cold tumors,[21] the SCNA level correlates with a poor treatment response (Ben-David and Amon, 2020; Knouse et al., 2017).

After several mutagenetic analyses of patient cohorts and cell line datasets, researchers found that one specific SCNA, the loss of chromosomal area 9p21.3, had a strong correlation with immune-cold tumors in head and neck cancers (Han et al., 2021; William et al., 2021). This association was particularly strong in tumors with rare mutations, which are present in a large majority of patients with advanced-stage head and neck cancers.

The 9p chromosomal region hosts many immune-regulating genes, said Davoli. How 9p-loss drives immune inactivation is not yet clear, but it could

---

[21] Immune-cold tumors are not likely to trigger a strong immune response due to their immune-suppressive tumor microenvironment and do not respond well to immunotherapy. See https://www.cancer.gov/publications/dictionaries/cancer-terms/def/cold-tumor (accessed May 11, 2023).

affect immune evasion via suppression of interferon pathways and signaling. Recent studies have suggested that chromosomal area 9p24 is strongly associated with the immune checkpoint blockade response and patient survival (Alhalabi et al., 2022; Spiliopoulou et al., 2022; Zhao et al., 2022).

Diagnostic Imaging

Marius Mayerhoefer, professor of radiology at Memorial Sloan Kettering Cancer Center, said that imaging, in combination with advances in measurement, modeling, and analytics, may soon provide a more holistic understanding of a patient's tumor, point to personalized treatments, and improve patient outcomes (see Figure 2). New imaging methods open opportunities to study new drug targets (Farwell et al., 2022; Guo et al., 2021; Kratochwil et al., 2019; Pandit-Taskar et al., 2022; Pereira et al., 2019; Vaz et al., 2020; Zhou et al., 2022). In addition, he noted that from a patient perspective, noninvasive imaging is preferred over multiple biopsies to monitor response.

Mayerhoefer said that although each technique has limitations and clinical trials are still lacking, imaging can offer advantages over biopsies by enabling a whole-body approach for understanding therapy response and assessing disease burden. For example, positron emission tomography (PET) scans provide functional and targeted imaging of cancer and immune cells, making them quantifiable. Radiomics approaches, which use mined data from imaging, can capture the heterogeneity of multiple tumors as opposed to single lesions.

Mayerhoefer said that a challenge with morphological imaging is distinguishing disease progression from pseudoprogression because decreases in tumor burden may not be evident until reimaging. PET imaging with the radionuclide fluorodeoxyglucose is well established for assessing tumor metabolic activity, but it cannot effectively distinguish between uptake by tumor versus immune cells. A novel PET method, immuno-PET,[22] can be used to radiolabel an antibody or an antibody fragment, or a small molecule, to better assess immune targets in the tumor (Jauw et al., 2017; Wei et al., 2018). Immuno-PET provides an opportunity for whole-body imaging of tumor burden and uptake of PD-1 expression (Bensch et al., 2018). Another method, contrast-enhanced magnetic resonance imaging (MRI), can also distinguish between tumor- and immune-related uptake and has been used to monitor tumor-associated macrophage responses to anti-CD47[23] immunotherapies (Mohanty et al., 2019a, 2019b).

---

[22] Immuno-PET uses both the PET imaging technique and the specificity of monoclonal antibody targeting, which enables noninvasive and very specific visualizations (Wei et al., 2020).

[23] CD47 is a surface protein important to distinguish healthy cells from old or diseased cells. Removal using anti-CD47 therapies would harness macrophage activity to attack cancerous cells. See https://med.stanford.edu/stemcell/CD47.html (accessed March 27, 2023).

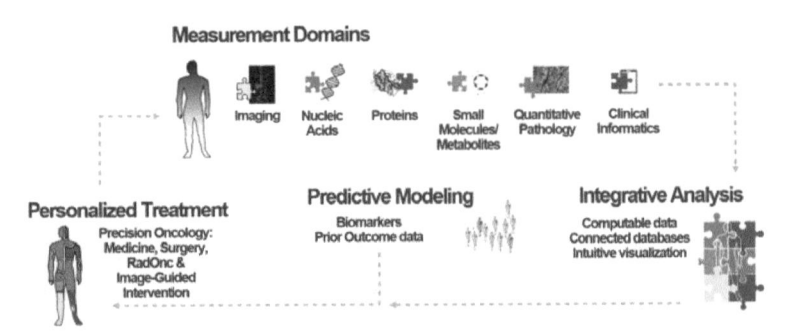

FIGURE 2 Conceptual diagram highlighting how imaging and other measurement domains provide a more holistic understanding of a patient's tumor to support integrative analysis, predictive modeling, and personalized treatment.
SOURCE: Mayerhoefer presentation, November 14, 2022.

Chris Boshoff, chief development officer of oncology and rare disease global product development at Pfizer Inc, asked how imaging addresses macrophage infiltration. Mayerhoefer answered that MRI with ferumoxytol can distinguish between M1 and M2 macrophages,[24] adding that pretreatment images should show more M2s, and imaging after a successful treatment should show more M1s for the antitumor effect, but this has not yet been proven.

In response to a question from Khleif, Mayerhoefer stated that his goal is to include more imaging in clinical trials and develop ways to see early response signals after one treatment cycle; clinical protocols specify certain imaging techniques, but he suggested that trials could move forward more quickly if they allowed for substituting a different technique.

Immune Metabolism

Hildegund Ertl, professor of vaccine and immunotherapy at the Wistar Institute, shared the results of her team's research into tumor metabolomics. Tumor vaccines, which aim to induce antigen-specific T cell-based cellular immunity to target tumor cells, can slow the progression of cancer, but over time, T cells lack nutrients, become exhausted, decline, and stop working. Tumor cells can also suffer from a lack of nutrients and become hypoglycemic when a tumor's glucose is depleted. When this lack of glucose is combined with hypoxia from low oxygen levels, tumors switch to fatty acid catabolism to survive (Zhang et al., 2017).

---

[24] M1 macrophages are generally proinflammatory and inhibit cell proliferation, whereas M2 macrophages are anti-inflammatory and linked to tissue repair (Yunna et al., 2020).

To test whether T cell survival could be enhanced, Ertl and her team vaccinated mice with an adenovirus vaccine that produces melanoma-associated antigen-specific CD8+ T cell response. The mice's tumors were then injected with fenofibrate, a drug that increases fatty acid metabolism, after which they saw a reduction in tumor progression and improvement in T cell function (Zhang et al., 2017). Even in vaccinated mice that were untreated with fenofibrate, researchers were able to force the tumor to switch from glycolysis to fatty acid catabolism, which made more glucose available for immune T cells, improving their function. Ertl's team found the same results in tumor fragments from humans transferred into mice and plan to recreate the switch to fatty acid catabolism when fenofibrate-treated tumor-infiltrating T cells are transferred into mice.

Novel Surrogate Biomarkers

Recent research into biomarkers for immune resistance is "mostly just at the tip of [the] iceberg," said W. Kimryn Rathmell, professor and chair of the Department of Medicine at Vanderbilt University Medical Center.[25] Most known biomarkers are tissue based, which often fail to capture the heterogeneity of the tumor, metastatic sites, and dormancy niches, making it difficult to create a complete picture of immunotherapy resistance. Rathmell said an ideal surrogate biomarker would provide information about the systemic disease state; be easily, rapidly, and repeatedly accessible via a minimally invasive modality; reliably quantify the immune and tumor response; and guide personalized successive treatment choices.

Imaging an immune response could help to identify surrogate biomarkers, such as glucose, said Rathmell. For example, fluorodeoxyglucose-PET scans can image cancer cells' uptake of glucose, which T cells also consume. Through studies across multiple tumor models, researchers discovered that it was not the T cells but the macrophages consuming the most glucose (specifically F18 glucose); cancer cells preferred F18 glutamine and were less inclined to consume fatty acids (Reinfeld et al., 2021). One important caveat is that immunotherapy can cause responses that make image interpretation difficult. To effectively identify biomarkers, imaging approaches need to visualize the tumor and distinguish among cancer cells, immune cells, and mixed signals, pointing to a need for improved imaging response or resistance indicators, Rathmell said.

Regulatory Considerations for Biomarkers in Cancer Immunotherapy

Reena Philip, associate director of biomarkers and precision oncology at the FDA Oncology Center of Excellence, discussed regulatory considerations

---

[25] Rathmell became director of the National Cancer Institute on December 18, 2023.

around immuno-oncology biomarkers. FDA-approved companion diagnostics related to immunotherapies include tumor PD-L1 expression, microsatellite instability-high (MSI-H)/deficient mismatch repair (dMMR), and tumor mutational burden-high (TMB-H).[26]

Philip explained that companion diagnostics are tests that provide information that is essential to safely and effectively use a corresponding therapeutic product, and these are included on the therapeutic label. Complementary diagnostics, in contrast, are tests that aid in risk-benefit assessments in patient care by identifying a biomarker-defined subset of patients who respond well to a particular therapy, but are not prerequisites for receiving the drug. The designation of companion versus complementary diagnostics is based on both the design and the outcomes of the clinical trials in which they were studied.

However, there is considerable variation even among companion diagnostics. For example, the four used for PD-L1 have different definitions of expression, cutoffs, and scoring, making standardization difficult; this led to a multistakeholder harmonization effort for these assays to enable comparisons across different antibodies, staining platforms, and clinical cutoffs (Hirsch et al., 2017; Tsao et al., 2018).

Philip also discussed opportunities and challenges in tissue-agnostic drug development. Immunotherapy was shown to be effective in treating patients whose tumors have dMMR (Le et al., 2015). In 2017, pembrolizumab was approved for treating tumors that test positive for MSI-H/dMMR, making it the first tissue-agnostic drug approval (Lemery et al., 2017). Pembrolizumab was then approved for treating TMB-H solid tumors in 2020. Philip noted that measurements for TMB using the companion diagnostic can have significant variability based on preanalytic conditions, analytic variables, and impacts from bioinformatics, which device manufacturers have attempted to harmonize through efforts with Friends of Cancer Research (Vega et al., 2021). For future efforts in tissue-agnostic drug development, Philip said that several factors need to be considered when determining whether a tissue-agnostic oncology drug development program may be scientifically and clinically appropriate. There are several challenges, including the low prevalence of a biomarker across tumor types, contributing to low sample size for each tumor type; enrollment challenges due to the rareness of biomarker in tumor type; having a clear definition of a biomarker and the cutoff for a tissue-agnostic indication; and lack of standardization of tests used across many different sites in global trials.

---

[26] MSI-H, dMMR, and TMB are biomarkers for cancer cells with a high number of mutations. See https://www.cancer.gov/publications/dictionaries/cancer-terms/def/microsatellite-instability-high-cancer; https://www.cancer.gov/publications/dictionaries/cancer-terms/def/mismatch-repair-deficiency; and https://www.cancer.gov/publications/dictionaries/cancer-terms/def/tumor-mutational-burden (accessed March 27, 2023).

Philip noted that many trials are also now evaluating circulating tumor DNA (ctDNA) as a biomarker for immunotherapy decision making, including trials of neoadjuvant therapy. Analysis of ctDNA could also potentially be used to predict response, evaluate mechanisms and genetic determinants of treatment resistance or response, differentiate between pseudoprogression and true progression, and decide when to switch therapies. Much is unknown about how best to use ctDNA assays, and, like other biomarkers, there is a need to standardize protocols, units of measurements, and assessments, she said.

Surrogate Endpoint Development

Nicole Gormley, director of the division of hematologic malignancies II and acting associate director for oncology endpoint development at the FDA Oncology Center of Excellence, discussed regulatory considerations around surrogate endpoint development. For regulatory use, such as patient stratification, selection, enrichment, or treatment, the Prentice Criteria state that the surrogate needs to be a correlate of the true clinical endpoint whose effect matches the full effect of treatment (Prentice, 1989). Because this criterion is quite strict, other validation methods have been developed via meta-analyses of patient- and trial-level data to determine the surrogate threshold effect, or the minimum treatment needed to predict a clinical benefit (Buyse et al., 2010; Sargent et al., 2015).

These methods have helped to identify several possible surrogate endpoints, Gormley said. In collaborative neoadjuvant trials for breast cancer, a pooled meta-analysis showed that an absence of residual invasive tumors in both the breast and axillary lymph nodes was associated with pathological complete response (pCR) and overall survival (Cortazar and Geyer, 2015). On an individual patient level, achieving pCR was associated with a reduced risk of death, suggesting that it could potentially be a surrogate endpoint (Cortazar et al., 2014). However, at the trial level, relatively little association appeared between pCR and death, and so pCR has not been approved as a surrogate endpoint. Another potential surrogate endpoint, also not yet approved, is minimal residual disease (MRD)[27] in multiple myeloma, which was identified after two trial-level meta-analyses showed that patients who were MRD negative, meaning no measurable disease was detected after treatment, had better overall survival rates (Landgren et al., 2016; Munshi et al., 2017).

Validated surrogate endpoints could expedite drug development, said Gormley. Although meta-analyses can be used to validate surrogate endpoints

---

[27] Measurable or minimal residual disease is a small number of cancer cells that remain in the body after treatment. This metric is used to measure treatment success and prognosis. See https://www.cancer.gov/publications/dictionaries/cancer-terms/def/mrd (accessed April 6, 2023).

for FDA approval, regulatory uncertainties remain, and Gormley noted that researchers should discuss with FDA the proposed use of novel surrogate endpoints in registration trials. She said that meta-analyses of surrogate endpoint development should consider data from multiple trials, with a wide range of effects, to improve statistical rigor and enable more interrogation of uncertainties; biomarker assessment timing; minimization of missing data; and ability to inform future applicability (Alonso et al., 2016; Buyse et al., 2010; Sargent and Mandrekar, 2013). The remaining challenges include how to ensure patient safety, demonstrate trial-level surrogacy, determine what threshold best correlates with clinical benefit, and identify the appropriate timing of assessment (FDA, 2019; Gormley et al., 2017).

Rathmell asked if FDA supported the use of more imaging tests, and Gormley replied that FDA can work with researchers to incorporate more imaging in clinical trials, noting that this information is important for building a comprehensive picture of the therapy being evaluated and the patient condition. Rathmell added that better clinical tools, including functional imaging, would enhance the overall understanding of immune activity: "I do not think we understand really what the basics of the human immune system are—what is normal?"

Fostering Collaboration

Luke asked how industry and academia can be better partners in biomarker development, noting that the MSI pathway was discovered through academic research but required industry backing to gain FDA approval. He said that the development of the TMB companion diagnostic was driven by industry, but pCR has languished without industry support. Boshoff answered that close collaboration among industry, academia, and FDA is needed. "Every time there is a success, it is when those three come together and actually deliver," he said. Davoli agreed, noting that biomarkers need to be developed into a companion diagnostic, which requires time and investment that companies are more likely to have.

Gormley and Theoret agreed that partnerships have been critical to the successes of immunotherapies. The return on investment for biomarker development may be lower than for drug development, Gormley added, but industry would still benefit from developing products that aid earlier disease detection, better response detection, and more efficient trial designs to expedite FDA approval. Boshoff noted that pembrolizumab and nivolumab development started in academia but had large industry-supported trials. He agreed that collaborative data sharing could enable researchers to revive shelved drug candidates and added that the nonprofit Friends of Cancer Research facilitates industry–academia collaboration and is open to research ideas. Boshoff also shared that Pfizer and FDA are collaborating with several large molecular profiling companies, sharing real-world data to generate evidence to validate surrogate endpoints.

Philip mentioned the Cancer Immune Monitoring and Analysis Center,[28] a network that was established to identify and assess new biomarkers, supporting immunotherapy clinical trials from NCI as well as from the Foundation for the National Institutes of Health's (FNIH's) Partnership for Accelerating Cancer Therapies. Theoret noted that FDA has a formal biomarker qualification program[29] for drug development tools to minimize patient risk and reminded participants that different datasets, such as meta-analyses, can be used to generate evidence to support drug development decisions.

Key Issues and Suggestions in Biomarkers and Surrogate Endpoints

Summarizing the discussions of biomarkers and surrogate endpoints, Rathmell and Boshoff pointed to many unanswered questions that hinder the advancement of immunotherapy development. How does a "normal" host-immune system work, and what is abnormal? How can the immune system be pushed into antitumor activity? How can a more holistic view of the tumor environment be obtained, in addition to biopsies? How can more effective imaging tools be incorporated into clinical care to determine treatment response? How does a tumor genome correspond to resistance? How can the validation process for biomarkers be streamlined?

THE ROLE OF DATA AND COMPUTATIONAL TOOLS

Regulatory and Access Considerations in Mining Big Data

Ahmad Tarhini, director of cutaneous clinical and translational research at the H. Lee Moffitt Cancer Center and Research Institute, highlighted opportunities to mine big data for scientific insights and described the regulatory and data access considerations involved in this approach. Large oncology datasets—including genomics, transcriptomics, epigenomics, proteomics, and metabolomics—have expanded dramatically in recent years, bringing new insights into the molecular basis of disease biology and host immunology. These data can be integrated with data from other sources, such as clinical trials, electronic health records (EHRs), bioimaging, and wearable sensors (Fröhlich et al., 2018).

Maintaining privacy of patients' data—today and in the future—is of paramount importance, said Tarhini. This requires continuing discussions to ensure all parties meet regulatory compliance, as governed by the Privacy Rule in the

---

[28] See https://cimac-network.org/ (accessed May 12, 2023).

[29] See https://www.fda.gov/drugs/drug-development-tool-ddt-qualification-programs/biomarker-qualification-program (accessed May 12, 2023).

United States and the General Data Protection Regulation in Europe, and continuous, thoughtful steps to share data responsibly, improve EHRs, and enhance patient consent and engagement, with an emphasis on reaching the global majority population, he said (Comandè and Schneider, 2018).

Tarhini said that one successful model of a data-sharing ecosystem is the Oncology Research Information Exchange Network (ORIEN), a collaboration to advance research via a common data collection protocol that maximizes regulatory compliance and data quality and compatibility while simplifying multisource data sharing. ORIEN's alliance, which includes cancer centers, clinicians, researchers, pharmaceutical and biotechnology companies, payers, and regulators, aims to serve and protect patients by following guiding principles of partnership, collaboration, inclusiveness, and accessibility to harmonized, aggregated, deidentified data. For example, ORIEN collaborations have advanced cancer research by demonstrating that signatures related to interferon gamma, effector T cells, chemokines, major histocompatibility complex Class II, and tertiary lymphoid structures were significantly predictive of ICI benefits for patients with melanoma (Tarhini et al., 2022).

Advanced Computing Tools

Jack Hidary, chief executive officer of SandboxAQ,[30] stated that quantum computing could open vast new opportunities to simulate molecular interactions, with the potential to revolutionize cancer drug discovery and development by lowering costs, times, toxicities, and failure rates. Quantum simulations are needed because the molecular interactions between antibodies and their targets entail electrons, which happens at the quantum level. "These are quantum chemical interactions," Hidary said. "We need to use the language of quantum physics to simulate this interaction."

Quantum computers do not yet exist, but quantum simulations are possible on classical computers (Ganahl et al., 2022; Hauru et al., 2021; Pederson et al., 2022). He said that fierce market competition has led to incredible advances in computer graphics processing units (GPU), a key computational platform for both quantum computing and AI. These advances enable modern computers to run large language models with billions of parameters, wide applicability, and powerful natural language processing (NLP)[31] abilities that can mine data from EHRs, journals, and other sources, assessing drug safety and efficacy much more quickly. Furthermore, applying ML techniques to real-world data sources will bring even more accuracy to these simulations, increasing the likelihood of quickly bringing new drugs to human trials and helping the many patients who

---

[30] See https://www.sandboxaq.com (accessed December 4, 2023).
[31] These computer systems can process human language (Nadkarni et al., 2011).

have yet to benefit from single-agent or combination immunotherapies, Hidary said.

Data-Driven Approaches for Modeling Response and Resistance

Pe'er described how modeling the complex cell and immune microenvironments using single-cell data can help researchers better understand immunotherapy resistance. Single-cell ribonucleic acid (RNA) sequencing has revealed that tumor microenvironments teem with undiscovered cell types (Laughney et al., 2020). Understanding that richness—and the potential for synergistic responses—has led to new therapeutic approaches, such as using expression of transcription factor 7[32] as a biomarker of ICI response or harnessing dendritic cells to enhance the immune response (Brown et al., 2019; Mayoux et al., 2020; Oh et al., 2020; Sade-Feldman et al., 2018). In another example, research on cells from the cerebrospinal fluid of patients with leptomeningeal metastases,[33] who face an extremely poor prognosis, demonstrated that the cancer cells expressed high levels of iron-binding proteins. A mouse model of leptomeningeal metastases showed that cancer cell growth could be inhibited by iron chelation therapy[34] (Chi et al., 2020). Based on these data, a pilot study in a small number of patients with leptomeningeal metastases demonstrated extended survival with this therapy.

Pe'er said that she does not typically think of single-cell data as "big data," because they often come from a small number of patients, but they are complex, with large matrices and millions of data points. To increase the sample sizes and achieve clinical covariates, Pe'er stressed the need to conduct meta-analyses from multiple clinical trials, facilitate data sharing, integrate different modalities, and infuse prior knowledge to fully understand the biology. As the expertise needed to integrate such data sources to model these complex interactions is relatively rare, Pe'er's team created an algorithm to examine cell type and gene signature data to quickly find interpretable gene programs using a Bayesian approach they call "Spectra factor analysis."[35]

---

[32] Transcription factors are proteins used during the process of transcribing DNA into RNA. See https://www.nature.com/scitable/definition/transcription-factor-167/ (accessed March 15, 2023).

[33] These cancers have spread to the protective membrane of the brain and spinal cord and/or the cerebrospinal fluid. See https://www.mskcc.org/cancer-care/patient-education/leptomeningeal-metastases (accessed March 28, 2023).

[34] Iron chelators reduce iron accumulation in cells. This can be used to combat cancer, as rapidly replicating cancerous cells need to metabolize more iron to continue growing (Ibrahim and O'Sullivan, 2020).

[35] For more information on Spectra, see the preprint manuscript at https://www.biorxiv.org/content/10.1101/2022.12.20.52131 (accessed March 28, 2023).

Spectra factor analysis enables entirely new discoveries by adapting to the data inputs; learning new factors; and incorporating prior knowledge, modeling, deep biological knowledge, and complex data tools. For example, researchers were able to distinguish between tumor-reactive and tumor-exhaustive T cells in breast cancer, making it possible to predict patient response to anti-PD-1 treatment (Bassez et al., 2021). Investigators also found a novel invasion factor in myeloid cells (Chan et al., 2021). "This, I think, is a really powerful approach of modeling it correctly, not only using the most powerful AI 'hammer' but thinking deeply," Pe'er said.

To continue this progress, Pe'er suggested that teams of immuno-oncology and computational experts should work together to craft more algorithms suited for single-cell and spatial data from well-designed cohorts, including responders and nonresponders, that can be aggregated and integrated with other modalities (Kunes et al., 2023). In addition, she said that several new spatial technologies, such as Lunaphore COMET,[36] iterative bleaching extends multiplexity,[37] 10x Visium,[38] and multiplexed error-robust fluorescence in situ hybridization,[39] can also be incorporated into studying cell–cell interactions and identify potential drug targets.

Leveraging Real-World Data to Characterize Immune-Related Adverse Events (irAEs)

Prakirthi Yerram, senior clinical director for research oncology real-world evidence at Flatiron Health, discussed how real-world data can be leveraged to understand irAEs, which affect a majority of patients and can range from minor to serious and even fatal (Esfahani et al., 2020). Studying irAEs can help researchers characterize their risk factors, such as the therapy timeline or patient age, although understanding causality remains challenging (Cathcart-Rake et al., 2020; Huang et al., 2021). Real-world data can help clinicians understand irAEs better and improve detection and management, although each data source has benefits and drawbacks.

Real-world data can come from many sources, including EHRs, pharmacovigilance, and health insurance claims. These sources often have larger sample

---

[36] For more information on the Lunaphore COMET, see https://lunaphore.com/products/comet/ (accessed March 28, 2023).

[37] A type of microscopy that uses iterative staining and bleaching to parse >65 parameters in a single tissue sample (Radtke et al., 2020).

[38] For more information on the 10X Genomics Visium CytAssist, see https://www.10xgenomics.com/instruments/visium-cytassist (accessed March 28, 2023).

[39] An imaging method that measures both RNA frequency and spatial distribution (Chen et al., 2015).

sizes and greater patient diversity than clinical trial data, with rich clinical detail. However, Yerram said that these data are often incomplete, and quality is highly variable. Access challenges and a lack of standardized reporting can also make it difficult to use and interpret these data sources, she noted.

Advances in ML and NLP are making it easier to extract information relevant to identifying irAEs from oncology EHR data, much of which is unstructured (e.g., clinician notes and hospitalization records) and highly time- and labor-intensive to process and characterize manually. For rare irAEs, Yerram said that ML and NLP techniques are likely to be especially helpful because integrating more real-world data sources can increase sample sizes. Standardizing irAE reporting to the FDA Adverse Event Reporting System[40] will also help to improve characterization.

AI, Data Science, and Big Data Approaches

Fayyad described how advanced digital approaches, such as AI, can have a large impact on health care by reducing costs; minimizing waste; and improving drug discovery, design, and effectiveness. For example, AI-empowered single-cell analytics, which enable real-time, direct observation of cell–cell interactions, could reduce the evaluation time for candidate therapies from months to days, he said.

For AI approaches to be effective, Fayyad said ML tools need to be trained on large sets of granular, high-quality data that are digital, extractable, structured, shareable, and manageable. These tools include NLP of data sources, image analysis techniques, graph-based and network representations, network science models for understanding multifactor interactions, and multi-omics approaches, which Fayyad said are especially promising in determining why patients with similar exomes or genomes may have dramatically different treatment responses.

Generating the necessary training data and fully incorporating these advances into processes for health care and life sciences research requires overcoming cultural resistance to change, Fayyad noted. AI approaches can be implemented incrementally, using test cases to build up a reference architecture. Also, a talented workforce of data and life sciences specialists is essential to creating complex, accurate algorithms and understanding their limitations, and an educational pipeline is needed to fill in this gap. Fayyad said that the Institute for Experiential Artificial Intelligence[41] focuses on taking on "real projects, with real data, for real organizations," emulating the residency model of medical school to

---

[40] See https://www.fda.gov/drugs/questions-and-answers-fdas-adverse-event-reporting-system-faers/fda-adverse-event-reporting-system-faers-public-dashboard (accessed December 4, 2023).

[41] See https://ai.northeastern.edu/ (accessed December 4, 2023).

gradually build the architecture and the staff needed to realize the potential of AI tools.

Fayyad also briefly described Northeastern's Observational Health Data Sciences and Informatics Center, a global open-source community creating and encouraging the use of common data models, such as the Observational Medical Outcomes Partnership,[42] to leverage these digital approaches for real-world evidence, such as long-term patient tracking in the United States and Europe.

Data Challenges

Julie Gralow, chief medical officer and executive vice president of the American Society of Clinical Oncology, asked panelists to name the biggest challenge in advanced computational techniques to find drivers of immune resistance. Yerram replied that the lack of data standardization, especially for pharmacovigilance elements, makes it difficult to effectively characterize and use data. Fayyad agreed, noting that systematically standardized and sharable data collection is the essential foundation to facilitating advanced computational methods. Leveraging AI for collecting publication data, for example, would be a large undertaking but could help researchers incorporate much more knowledge into future research efforts. "The good news is that it is solvable," Fayyad said. "The bad news is that it requires effort to get it done." Pe'er and Tarhini agreed that achieving standardized data and collection protocols is a Herculean task, requiring experts skilled in working with the existing imperfect data. Pe'er said that new AI tools developed for the coronavirus disease of 2019 (COVID-19), such as AlphaFold's building blocks,[43] have demonstrated that AI can accelerate drug design.

When Rathmell asked what an "ideal" dataset looks like, Pe'er said that it depends on the research question, but large-scale data standardization is possible. For example, Israel and the United Kingdom have a standardized EHR system. Noting that EHRs are currently too heterogeneous to be a good source of data worldwide, Fayyad suggested that a global system, driven by use cases and standardized to eliminate variances, is needed (Shull, 2019). Tarhini posited that existing industry collaborations between real-world evidence companies, such as ConcertAI,[44] and EHR vendors could model better data collection and sharing techniques.

---

[42] The Observational Medical Outcomes Partnership worked to improve health care databases that recorded medical device use outcomes. For more information, see https://ohdsi.org/omop/ (accessed May 16, 2023).

[43] AlphaFold is an AI tool developed by DeepMind to predict 3-D models of protein structures. For further information, see https://www.deepmind.com/research/highlighted-research/alphafold (accessed March 28, 2023).

[44] See https://www.concertai.com/ (accessed March 28, 2023).

Diana Vega, director of oncology and translational medicine strategy at AstraZeneca, pointed out that researchers cannot be expected to know future research questions and may unwittingly collect incomplete or too much data, creating storage and cost issues. Fayyad replied that to combat this, researchers can start with questions for very specific use cases, undergone one at a time, to guide specific data collection, management, and storage requirements while creating a reference architecture that can be used in the future. Nancy Davidson, executive vice president of clinical affairs, senior vice president, and professor in the clinical research division at Fred Hutchinson Cancer Center, added that cost and patient security are of critical importance. Tarhini noted that ORIEN, which is funded by pharmaceutical companies and has a commercial arm, facilitates the exchange of all types of data for researchers asking specific questions.

Gralow asked about the role for Minimal Common Oncology Data Elements (mCODE), which is a collaboration among clinicians, scientists, FDA, and EHR manufacturers to increase the amount of high-quality, shareable data available to clinicians and researchers to support patient care (Osterman et al., 2020). It has attempted to standardize terms in EHRs and clinical trials and is testing use cases to determine efficacy. "We need standardization, and we need structured data," said Lawrence Shulman, professor of medicine at the Perelman School of Medicine, associate director for special projects at the Abramson Cancer Center, and director of the Center for Global Cancer Medicine at the University of Pennsylvania. Tarhini and Fayyad emphasized that continued use and evolution are the best way to grow such standards.

Patient-Reported Data

Jeannine Brant, board president of the Oncology Nursing Society, asked how data from electronic patient-reported outcomes, devices or applications that capture much of the patient experience but lack processing and analysis workflows, might be better leveraged to aid in these efforts. Fayyad replied that these excel at collecting critical data but are unstructured. Collecting structured—and therefore usable—data is the goal but is often prohibitively expensive. Tarhini suggested that a collaboration between ORIEN researchers and device makers could help.

Addressing Bias

Gwen Darien, executive vice president of patient advocacy and engagement at the National Patient Advocate Foundation, asked how to address bias in data collection to ensure that these new digital tools promote health equity for all instead of perpetuating inequities. For example, race and ancestry standards evolve as our historical understanding does. Yerram replied that Flatiron, like the AI field as a whole, is trying to understand the potential biases in its algorithms before validating them for predictive uses, especially for patient demographics. Fayyad added that audits should systematically detect and assess unintended biases.

Key Issues and Suggestions for Data and Computational Tools

Reflecting on the session's discussions, Gralow and Davidson highlighted several challenges and opportunities to advance progress. First, there is a need to better characterize immunotherapy response, resistance, and irAEs. Second, there is a lack of data standardization, and there are issues with data quality, quantity, security, sharing, patient privacy, and regulatory compliance. Finally, a number of speakers underscored the need for better communication among researchers, clinicians, and patients.

Many speakers offered suggestions for improving immunotherapy research, including adopting advanced computing tools and quantum molecular models, investigating single-cell data, standardizing and structuring data elements (similar to mCODE, and especially in EHRs), improving ML and NLP abilities for unstructured data, and incentivizing data sharing and communication. Davidson said that it will be important to train the next generation of investigators to be fluent across disciplines, including biology, medicine, data science, and AI.

CRITERIA TO ASSESS CANCER IMMUNOTHERAPY COMBINATIONS IN EARLY-PHASE CLINICAL TRIALS: TRIAL DESIGNS FOR REGULATORY APPROVAL

Novel Clinical Trial Designs

Keith Flaherty, director of clinical research at Massachusetts General Hospital Cancer Center and professor of medicine at Harvard Medical School, stated that new clinical trial strategies, especially at the early stages, are needed to demonstrate proof of concept and pull immunotherapy out of what he described as this "disappointingly unproductive time."

First, he suggested that publicly funded clinical trials should be allowed to use existing biomarker data to rapidly identify patients who are unlikely to respond to the single-agent standard of care and switch them to investigational treatments, such as anti-LAG-3 or a combination of anti-CTLA-4 with anti-PD-1 (Lipson et al., 2021; Wolchok et al., 2021). In addition, he stressed that researchers should not only investigate fully refractory patients but also begin using adaptive strategies to find patients who may have a stable outcome or delayed response to investigational therapy. For example, novel immunologic response assessment tools, such as imaging, plasma proteomics, and biomarkers from biopsies, can more quickly determine the efficacy of novel agents and shed light on resistance mechanisms. By performing single-cell RNA sequencing on serial tumor biopsies of patients with melanoma receiving anti-PD-1 therapy, researchers have been able to distinguish markers of response and nonresponse and accurately predict outcomes at a far earlier point (Chen et al., 2016; Sade-Feldman et al., 2018).

Ex vivo functional diagnostics, which examine tumor–immune interactions in tumor explants, can also shed light on resistance mechanisms, and research has shown that the tumor explant's response correlates with patient response to the immunotherapy (Jenkins et al., 2018; Sehgal et al., 2021). Flaherty posited that these diagnostics could also be used for investigational therapeutic decision making. In addition, approaches in which an in vivo injected device pumps out microdoses of investigational therapies have shown promise (Jonas et al., 2015).

Public–Private Partnerships

Roy Herbst, Ensign Professor of Medicine and professor of pharmacology, chief of medical oncology, and associate director for translational research at Yale Cancer Center and Yale School of Medicine, highlighted how public–private partnerships can leverage and share resources and knowledge, diversify clinical trials, and advance innovation for the benefit of patients. He said that trials supported through these partnerships are most efficient and successful when master protocols[45] are used to ensure smooth implementation, oversight, conduct, and monitoring. This requires detailed planning, communication, specification and an emphasis on teamwork, innovation, and flexibility within constraints. He emphasized that trials should also be science driven, patient focused, diverse, and translational.

One FNIH initiative, the Lung Cancer Master Protocol (LungMAP), is an NCI-led collaboration of clinicians and drug manufacturers on a set of large, open, multiarm, biomarker-driven, single-agent and combination clinical trials for diverse patients with all lung cancer types, including refractory cancers, with no-cost screening that connects patients at more than 700 clinics with the appropriate trial (Malik et al., 2014). Several elements have contributed to its success, Herbst said. First, it has strong governance and oversight. Second, the trials can evolve with the treatment landscape. Third, the partners developed cohesive project management and thoughtful approaches to drug selection, study design, prescreening, patient diversity, and practices to translate the findings—in mutations,

---

[45] A master protocol is a design infrastructure in which one protocol can comprise a variety of studies that examine multiple different therapies (multiarm) or multiple subpopulations. For master protocol design information, see https://www.fda.gov/media/120721/download (accessed March 29, 2023). For further information on LungMAP, see https://www.lung-map.org/about-lung-map (accessed March 13, 2023).

biomarkers, liquid biopsies, and multi-omics profiling—into the standard of care for lung cancers that have been very difficult to treat. For example, patients given a novel combination of ICI (pembrolizumab) with vascular endothelial growth factor inhibition had a significant improvement in survival compared to the standard of care (Reckamp et al., 2022). "This is team science at its best," Herbst said.

Assessing the Contributions of Individual Components

Theoret discussed approaches to assess the contributions of individual components in the context of combination immunotherapies. PD-1 inhibitors are part of the first-line standard of care as a monotherapy or in combination for numerous types of cancer (Upadhaya et al., 2022), yet immunotherapy response patterns of anti-PD-1 therapy, such as pseudoprogression, lesion reduction, or stability, suggest meaningful patient endpoints only when the trial population is properly characterized, which has posed a challenge (Blumenthal et al., 2017; Mulkey et al., 2020; Wolchok et al., 2009). To overcome this challenge, multidisciplinary groups have tried to minimize the likelihood of a late or poor response by clearly defining a resistant population by studying dose exposure, response before disease progression, and potential for late progression.

For combination therapies with anti-PD-1, this process is more complicated. To ensure patient safety but still enable flexibility, FDA requires that trials demonstrate the contribution of effect (COE) for a fixed dosage of each individual agent used in combination therapies. Randomized controlled trials generate the best COE evidence, especially for patients whose cancers are PD-1 resistant; without such data, researchers can use relevant external evidence to compare efficacy and endpoints, although doing so increases uncertainty for novel drugs or combinations. External evidence may include a strong biological rationale, safety and efficacy demonstrated in other indications, or data indicating that a monotherapy is minimally active.

Theoret shared several trial designs that could demonstrate COE, even with immune-resistant patients, such as a multiarm trial for each monotherapy and add-on designs. He also encouraged clinicians to refer to relevant FDA resources (FDA, 2013). Given the lack of a formal definition of resistance and the limited knowledge about resistance mechanisms, FDA recommends that patient eligibility criteria be tailored to the enrolling population and that overall response rate or a similar long-term measure demonstrating some clinical benefit be used as an endpoint to fully capture COE (FDA, 2013; Kluger et al., 2020).

NCI Perspective

Sharon stated that with the right design, adaptive and multiarm clinical trials of early-stage combination therapy can be successful, even resulting in FDA approval. He provided an example of what he described as an ideal trial design for testing a combination of two active agents (see Figure 3) and noted that it has been used to study a combination of a PD-1 inhibitor with olaparib (an inhibitor of poly ADP ribose polymerase) for breast cancer. However, progress has been hindered by a limited understanding of—and tools to overcome—various resistance mechanisms, such as T cell immunosuppression,[46] a lack of T cell response, tumoral barriers to T cell infiltration, and issues with antigen presentation[47] (Day et al., 2017).

Patients with specific mutations or sensitivities may initially respond to immunotherapy treatments, but that response often does not represent a cure, so novel experimental combinations may be warranted. He said that data from single-arm combination trials are often inadequate to assess novel combinations (Foster et al., 2020), but as Theoret explained, multiple potential designs exist for efficient, randomized, multiarm combination trials to compare both single-agent and combination activity, demonstrate patient benefit (even with previously resistant tumors), and use interim analyses to eliminate trial arms or stop trials early if no benefit is detected. "By essentially taking account of the potential for success and the potential for failure at every stage, you can gain information with every single patient that you enroll," Sharon said.

Many speakers stressed that validated biomarkers are critical for immunotherapy drug development, and Sharon cautioned against using experimental, unvalidated biomarkers in trials. During clinical trial development, Sharon said

---

[46] T cell immunosuppression is carried out by a subset of CD4+ helper T cells called "regulatory T cells." They are responsible for ensuring the immune system does not attack the body's cells (self-tolerance) but can also suppress anti-cancer functions (Togashi et al., 2019).

[47] Antigen presentation is when molecules are presented on certain immune cells to aid in targeting. This helps other immune cells identify healthy versus unhealthy cells (i.e., infected, cancerous, senescent). When this process does not work properly, cancerous cells are not properly targeted by the immune system (Jhunjhunwala et al., 2021).

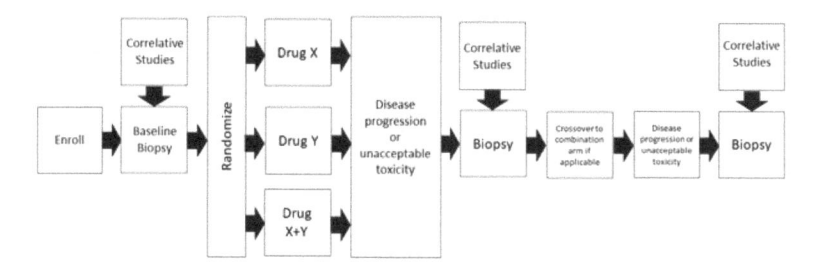

FIGURE 3 Clinical trial design for combination studies with two active agents.
SOURCES: Sharon presentation, November 15, 2022; Sharon and Foster, 2023.

researchers should identify potential biomarkers and determine whether they are relevant to either patient eligibility or endpoints.

Industry Perspective

Alexandra Snyder, chief medical officer at Generate Biomedicines and previous head of translational oncology at Merck, offered an industry perspective on how to approach clinical trial failures and ways to increase rates of success. Despite good early clinical evidence, plenty of phase III trials still fail (Diab et al., 2022; Hurwitz et al., 2019; Long et al., 2019; Mitchell et al., 2018). Snyder said these failures not only cause economic losses for the companies involved but can also encourage other companies to end similar drug trials early so as to avoid unnecessary losses. Failed late-stage trials show that success is not always possible, even with realistic and accurate modeling of a drug's features, dosing, patient selection, and other considerations. Snyder said that it is important to minimize the ripple effects from failed clinical trials, especially for smaller biotechnology companies, which are more likely to originate novel experimental drugs but also operate under tremendous financial pressures, creating a barrier to the field's advancement. She also suggested that it should be standard practice to publish translational research from failed studies.

Failed trials raise many questions. Could the study have used biomarkers to identify the patients most likely to benefit? How can drugs move forward with limited preclinical data? Can companies be incentivized to study failures? The high rate of failure among oncology trials underscores the urgent need to address these questions, Snyder said. She added that it is important to recognize how all of this fits into the difficult strategic decisions that pharmaceutical companies make, including decisions such as whether to focus on one drug or diversify their investments, the appropriate level of investment needed, and the current market dynamics.

To improve trial success rates, Snyder suggested that clinicians should define a biologically effective dose, or even randomize doses early on, instead of using the traditional maximum tolerated dose (Lancet Oncology, 2018; Shah et al., 2021). She also highlighted the need to diversify combinations, which is already occurring in the field (Upadhaya et al., 2022). She said that biotech companies could also diversify risk, randomize early, reevaluate response metrics, collaborate more, exercise restraint when other companies succeed or fail, and pivot away from combinations that only involve immunotherapies by adding other therapeutic mechanisms in combination trials. Finally, more judicious use of tools such as pharmacodynamics markers, surrogate biomarkers, and modeling could enable smaller, more nimble trials that still demonstrate activity.

Incorporating Pharmacodynamics

Jedd Wolchok, Meyer Director of the Sandra and Edward Meyer Cancer Center and professor of medicine at Weill Cornell Medicine, said that in many cases, it may not be that a drug failed but that the trial was not designed appropriately to measure success. For example, trials with the CTLA-4 blocker ipilimumab showed both conventional and novel response patterns. The novel patterns, pseudoprogression and the appearance of new lesions, were obstacles to assessing therapeutic response, even though patients showed a better survival rate with ipilimumab than with chemotherapy, albeit a very small number of patients (Chapman et al., 1999; Leach et al., 1996; Schadendorf et al., 2015). Patients with these novel responses still experienced long-term regression, making the standard clinical trial metric of progression-free survival at 12 weeks unsuitable (Wolchok et al., 2008).

To create new metrics, clinicians are turning to new modalities, such as immuno-PET, to find new pharmacodynamics endpoints, such as a tumor's T cell count, to predict outcome (Pandit-Taskar et al., 2022). He said that second-generation drugs may not cause tumor regression and should not necessarily be abandoned—measuring pharmacodynamic activity can also demonstrate immune activation, even if no tumor regression is apparent. For example, researchers have ended clinical trials of treatments targeting glucocorticoid-induced tumor-necrosis-factor-related (GITR) genes,[48] which were designed to overcome immunotherapy resistance, due to lack of tumor regression (Watts, 2005). But, if the goal had been to demonstrate pharmacodynamic activity (a decrease in the number of regulatory T cells), the results would have been viewed very differently.

In another example, the anti-GITR agent DTA-1 decreased tumors' regulatory T cells in mice. In humans, a promising pharmacodynamic marker showed that despite little antitumor activity, the drug did modulate its target (Cohen et al., 2010; Zappasodi et al., 2019). A subsequent trial with a combination of anti-PD-1 and anti-GITR therapies showed antitumor activity, although this study was prematurely ended due to financial difficulties (Davar et al., 2022).

Biomarkers for Early-Phase Trials

Herbst asked panelists to comment on the role of biomarkers in moving from early- to late-phase trials. Flaherty replied that the key challenge is that early-stage trials of investigational therapies will not have the validated response

---

[48] GITR activation has been found to modulate activity of different types of T cells to promote anti-tumor effects (Buzzatti et al., 2020).

biomarkers associated with clinical benefit, making it difficult to predict benefit. Therefore, novel drugs present necessary risks, and novel modalities, such as immuno-PET or ctDNA, can be used to find new biomarkers to support later-phase trials, which are longer and more expensive.

Sharon agreed, noting that although the workshop speakers mentioned many promising potential biomarkers, many of these are still unvalidated surrogates, and until they are correlated with clinically meaningful data, they cannot be used to predict outcomes. He said the RECIST criteria are validated as a surrogate of patient benefit and speculated that they will be used until something better is created and validated.

Snyder characterized three types of biomarkers in phase I trials—patient selection, response to treatment, and patient benefit—that can demonstrate proof of concept and help patients sooner. Theoret added that patient selection biomarkers can be incorporated into trial stratification. Response biomarkers, on the other hand, can be used to assess pharmacodynamic target engagement or dose selection or validate surrogate endpoints to predict clinical effect, but their use in clinical trials can increase the risk to patients. Thus, it is important to determine their correlation to clinically meaningful outcomes.

Wolchok suggested that phase I trials should have fewer expectations, enroll more patients, and have more time to allow the data to mature before an investigational agent's clinical value is assessed. Their outcomes should also be recast to determine whether a drug caused the immune response predicted from preclinical data before "abandoning an entire class of drugs," he said. Once identified, a mechanistic biomarker could assess whether the drug hit its target, making it easier to identify the relevant patient population and move to phase II trials, alone or in combination. Herbst added that determining criteria to move from phase II to phase III trials can also be challenging (Atkins et al., 2022).

Using and Sharing Data and Samples

Rathmell asked about guidelines for sharing biomarker samples. Sharon replied that data from NCI and the National Clinical Trials Network are a public resource accessible to researchers. Herbst said the same of LungMAP and speculated that many similar public resources are underused and should be more widely promoted, perhaps through policies that encourage sample lending in addition to banking.

Lippman asked about privately held anonymized samples or data from big pharmaceutical clinical trials, and Snyder replied that different companies have different approaches; at Merck, investigators can apply to view retrospective data, although such requests are subject to relevant regulations and company rules. The bigger challenge is translating retrospective findings prospectively. However, some companies are moving toward doing their own translational retrospective analyses.

When asked about opportunities to learn from failed studies, Snyder replied that time and expense are the main obstacles, although sample sizes can also be insufficient. However, these retrospective analyses could turn failed drugs into successes, and she suggested they become a study requirement. Herbst noted that public–private partnerships could examine the results of failed trials for useful data on response, disease stability, and potential biomarkers. Sharon agreed, noting that FDA's Project Optimus established dosage recommendations for some oncology drugs; NCI, FNIH, and other partners could incentivize a similar collaboration, minimizing the financial risks on the part of industry.

Key Issues and Suggestions on Criteria to Assess Immunotherapy Combinations in Early-Phase Clinical Trials

Herbst and Hedvig Hricak, Carroll and Milton Petrie Chair of the Department of Radiology at Memorial Sloan Kettering Cancer Center, professor of radiology at Weill Medical College of Cornell University, and professor of molecular pharmacology at Gerstner Sloan Kettering Graduate School of Biomedical Sciences, described several key issues from the session. First, negative clinical trial results can have dramatic repercussions for the entire field. Second, validated biomarkers for patient selection, immune response, and outcome are crucial to development and would be a dramatic improvement over RECIST. Third, phase I trials are for data interpretation, not extrapolation. Fourth, early randomized designs are preferable to single-arm trials for demonstrating the COE for components of combination therapies. Finally, regulatory requirements are best met through multidisciplinary collaborations, public–private partnerships, and communication with FDA.

They also summarized suggestions to advance the field. First, a number of participants suggested that public–private partnerships should be incentivized to encourage large-scale, collaborative clinical trials of combination therapies. Second, trial designs could be improved by enabling broader patient access to enhance diversity; ensuring that clinical endpoints are evaluated and analyzed for correlation with any predictive biomarkers; enhancing biomarker development and validation strategies; leveraging new methodologies, such as ex vivo and in vivo functional diagnostics; incorporating pharmacodynamic activity; randomizing dosing to find the biologically effective dose; and identifying patients to triage with first-line investigational therapies. Herbst said that clinicians should be able to add novel agents to the standard of care if a patient experiences suboptimal response. "Very complicated trials using technologies that are going to take teams of investigators, innovative trial designs, [and] adaptive approaches—I think that's going to be the future, to really pull all these pieces together and to do smarter trials, faster trials, and collaborative trials," said Herbst.

REFLECTIONS AND SUGGESTIONS TO ADDRESS TREATMENT RESISTANCE AND IMPROVE THE DEVELOPMENT OF IMMUNE MODULATOR THERAPEUTICS

Weiner and Lippman moderated a closing discussion to highlight opportunities to advance progress in understanding treatment resistance and to improve immune modulator therapeutic development.

Current Challenges and Possible Solutions

Session moderators summarized current challenges in immunotherapy resistance, along with possible solutions to enable a more holistic view of the tumor environment and advance the development of new therapies. Khleif and Weiner said that key problems include suboptimal clinical trial designs; a lack of understanding of resistance and its mechanisms, tumor response, and "normal" immune function; and inadequate data collection and analysis. A wide range of possible solutions were suggested.

First, Khleif said that workshop discussions indicated that preclinical models are crucial to improve clinical trial results because they can help determine an agent's mechanisms of action, response, and resistance before phase I trials; understand its COE; identify potential combination treatments; and identify and develop biomarkers, which are essential to aid patient selection and predict immune response.

Second, he said that updated clinical trial designs need be randomized, adaptive, and multiarm (enabling triaging with investigational therapies). Khleif said that trials also need clearly defined endpoints; the incorporation of new modalities, such as imaging and functional diagnostics; and broadened patient access for improved diversity.

Third, Weiner said that workshop sessions highlighted the need for improvements in data standardization, structure, quality, quantity, security, regulatory compliance, and sharing, to both enhance traditional research strategies and better leverage the capabilities of advanced computational tools. Finally, he emphasized that multidisciplinary collaboration and communication, as exemplified in public–private partnerships, are essential to encourage the cross-disciplinary learning necessary to accomplish these goals.

Defining Dosages

When asked if large, randomized trials to test different doses are practical to conduct, Blumenthal replied that they are more efficient in demonstrating preliminary evidence of clinical signals, such as biomarkers, pharmacokinetic and pharmacodynamic activity, dosage response, and safety. This information can then be used to determine the optimal dosage of a promising drug or combination. Theoret added that Project Optimus is focused on premarket drug characterization and dose optimization, a shift from traditional chemotherapy trials that focused on finding the maximum tolerated dose. Early-stage trials are streamlined to evaluate not only dose optimization but also pharmacodynamic and pharmacokinetic activity, safety, tolerability, and efficacy data. These metrics are correlated with patient outcomes to find suitable dose ranges and intervals to carry into a clinical trial. Postmarket dose optimization, on the other hand, is challenging, expensive, and often not beneficial to patients, Theoret noted.

Biomarker Development

Boshoff named surrogate endpoint biomarkers as the most important concept emerging from the workshop, especially for optimal dose selection. Unfortunately, finding them is not a simple task. He stated that advancing them will require securely sharing large databases across industry, academia, and FDA. In addition, Boshoff stressed that clinical trials have to be extremely robust, and tissue-based biomarkers from small, nonrandomized, or single-arm trials are unreliable and unlikely to be relevant across cancers. However, they can be used to analyze a subpopulation with a certain biomarker, such as 9p21 loss, to find primary or secondary endpoints, as occurred in phase III trials of renal and bladder cancer, which collected samples for RNA sequencing, epigenetic analyses, and proteomics to identify biomarkers (Larkin et al., 2022; Powles et al., 2023). In his view, the biggest challenge is using biomarkers to identify patients who do *not* need combination therapy or even immunotherapy.

Lippman asked whether drugs that do not meet their endpoints should be abandoned, even if a promising biomarker was found in a small set of patients. In that case, Boshoff replied, the drug would not be abandoned, and although it would not necessarily be approved by FDA, it could point to the need for a new trial for that patient subgroup. Pharmaceutical companies are interested in developing biomarkers, he stressed, even for small subsets of patients, because trials with the right biomarker are more likely to be successful, providing valuable information for the field and financial rewards for the company. Hricak added that the field needs more standardization for developing and validating biomarkers, especially in the preclinical phase.

Identifying Game-Changers

Fayyad and Weiner asked participants to name game-changing ideas that emerged during workshop presentations and discussions. Weiner began by stating that researchers need to do more than "admire the problem." He identified three ideas: design trials to facilitate learning from failure, make trials more efficient, and reach consensus on data collection and treatment guidelines for intralesional therapy. Blumenthal suggested that NCI could create a committee to thoroughly study failed trials.

Given the clear interest in making trials more pragmatic, Rathmell suggested that industry, regulators, and clinical investigators should collaborate on new designs, including for biomarker identification and validation. Gralow said that the rapid transitions to telehealth during the COVID-19 pandemic were challenging but also created new opportunities for conducting more pragmatic trials. Gralow, Theoret, and Lippman noted that telework and telehealth technologies make decentralized clinical trials easier, which increases trial participation, diversity, and patient convenience and allows researchers to design trials that are simpler and more flexible.

Theoret added that Project Optimus can be a model for other groups to capitalize on new insights into drug safety and tolerability. He also agreed that greater multisector collaboration would move the field forward efficiently and demonstrate the COE for biomarker-driven patient populations, noting that "none of us is stronger than all of us."

Davidson highlighted the adoption of universal data standards and appropriate biomedical and data science training for the next generation of clinical investigators as game-changing ideas. She added that investigators should be as well trained in computational tools as they are in biology and medicine. Khleif agreed that current researchers should also be trained in AI and other advanced computational techniques and use these tools to derive new conclusions from existing data. Khleif and Rathmell added that it is important train as many people as possible in clinical trial work and data science.

Tawbi pointed to the need to better understand resistance to immunotherapies, which requires measuring, quantifying, and targeting it; identifying patients who will experience it; and characterizing the drugs under development to understand whether it can be overcome. He noted that he is part of a collaboration to access and analyze data from thousands of clinical trials to understand and define the clinical phenotypes of resistance (Kluger et al., 2020), although it faced headwinds in its efforts to facilitate sharing of large-scale, privately held clinical trial data. He emphasized that these data can and should be shared safely to enable more rational drug development. Building on this point, Khleif said that large pharmaceutical companies' unwillingness to share their data represents a major obstacle; overcoming this reluctance might require new laws and policies incentivizing data sharing, minimizing companies' risks, and protecting their intellectual property. He said that precedents exist, in the computing and airline industries and pursuit of the COVID-19 vaccine, but it is nevertheless a daunting task.

Blumenthal mentioned successful initiatives, such as Project Data Sphere,[49] to share legacy (or "cold") data from clinical trials, which poses less risk for companies, but agreed that incentivizing companies to share more recent data would require legislative changes. Boshoff pointed out that Pfizer has approved many data-sharing requests in the hopes of finding and validating surrogate endpoint biomarkers, such as with Project FrontRunner,[50] and although these data are highly sought after, they may not be as valuable as some think. Tawbi asked if cold data were worth analyzing, and Lippman replied that care is needed to avoid data misuse, but safe sharing of genomic data can be a game changer for biomarker development. He also suggested that researchers should look at how other industries and medical fields are safely sharing data.

Khleif stated that to put game-changing ideas into action and solve the problems crystallized in this workshop, the next step is to influence and adopt regulatory changes that make it easier to safely move novel agents and combinations into clinical trials. Gralow agreed, adding that clinical trials need to be more pragmatic, decentralized, patient centric, and broadly eligible to create widely applicable results. And, although much of the conversation was about combination therapies, she stressed that some patients need less therapy, not more. Meanwhile, on a global scale, most patients lack any access to immunotherapy. "Don't forget about the rest of the world," she cautioned. "We're talking about science here and a lot of exciting stuff, but if we could just get these [existing] drugs to the whole world, we would be saving tens of thousands of lives tomorrow."

REFERENCES

Abou-El-Enein, M., M. Elsallab, S. A. Feldman, A. D. Fesnak, H. E. Heslop, P. Marks, B. G. Till, G. Bauer, and B. Savoldo. 2021. Scalable manufacturing of CAR T cells for cancer immunotherapy. *Blood Cancer Discovery* 2(5):408–422.

Alhalabi, O., J. Chen, Y. Zhang, Y. Lu, Q. Wang, S. Ramachandran, R. S. Tidwell, G. Han, X. Yan, J. Meng, R. Wang, A. G. Hoang, W. L. Wang, J. Song, L. Lopez, A. Andreev-Drakhlin, A. Siefker-Radtke, X. Zhang, W. F. Benedict, A. Y. Shah, J. Wang, P. Msaouel, M. Zhang, C. C. Guo, B. Czerniak, C. Behrens, L. Soto, V. Papadimitrakopoulou, J. Lewis, W. Rinsurongkawong, V. Rinsurongkawong, J. Lee, J. Roth, S. Swisher, I. Wistuba, J. Heymach, J. Wang, M. T. Campbell, E. Efstathiou, M. Titus, C. J. Logothetis, T. H. Ho, J. Zhang, L. Wang, and J. Gao. 2022. MTAP deficiency creates an exploitable target for antifolate therapy in 9p21-loss cancers. *Nature Communications* 13(1):1797.

Alonso, A., W. Van der Elst, G. Molenberghs, M. Buyse, and T. Burzykowski. 2016. An information-theoretic approach for the evaluation of surrogate endpoints based on causal inference. *Biometrics* 72(3):669–677.

---

[49] See https://www.projectdatasphere.org/ (accessed March 28, 2023).

[50] See https://www.fda.gov/about-fda/oncology-center-excellence/project-frontrunner (accessed March 28, 2023).

Amaria, R. N., M. Postow, E. M. Burton, M. T. Tezlaff, M. I. Ross, C. Torres-Cabala, I. C. Glitza, F. Duan, D. R. Milton, K. Busam, L. Simpson, J. L. McQuade, M. K. Wong, J. E. Gershenwald, J. E. Lee, R. P. Goepfert, E. Z. Keung, S. B. Fisher, A. Betof-Warner, A. N. Shoushtari, M. Callahan, D. Coit, E. K. Bartlett, D. Bello, P. Momtaz, C. Nicholas, A. Gu, X. Zhang, B. R. Korivi, M. Patnana, S. P. Patel, A. Diab, A. Lucci, V. G. Prieto, M. A. Davies, J. P. Allison, P. Sharma, J. A. Wargo, C. Ariyan, and H.A. Tawbi. 2022. Neoadjuvant relatlimab and nivolumab in resectable melanoma. *Nature* 611(7934):155–160.

Andrews, L. P., A. R. Cillo, L. Karapetyan, J. M. Kirkwood, C. J. Workman, and D. A. Vignali. 2022. Molecular pathways and mechanisms of LAG3 in cancer therapy. *Clinical Cancer Research* 28(23):5030–5039.

Atkins, M. B., H. Abu-Sbeih, P. A. Ascierto, M. R. Bishop, D. S. Chen, M. Dhodapkar, L. A. Emens, M. S. Ernstoff, R. L. Ferris, T. F. Greten, J. L. Gulley, R. S. Herbst, R. W. Humphrey, J. Larkin, K. A. Margolin, L. Mazzarella, S. S. Ramalingam, M. M. Regan, B. I. Rini, and M. Sznol. 2022. Maximizing the value of Phase III trials in immuno-oncology: A checklist from the Society for Immunotherapy of Cancer (SITC). *Journal for ImmunoTherapy of Cancer* 10(9):e005413.

Bashyam, H. 2007. CTLA-4: From conflict to clinic. *Journal of Experimental Medicine* 204(6):1243.

Bassez, A., H. Vos, L. Van Dyck, G. Floris, I. Arijs, C. Desmedt, B. Boeckx, M. Vanden Bempt, I. Nevelsteen, K. Lambein, K. Punie, P. Neven, A. D. Garg, H. Wildiers, J. Qian, A. Smeets, and D. Lambrechts. 2021. A single-cell map of intratumoral changes during anti-PD1 treatment of patients with breast cancer. *Nature Medicine* 27(5):820–832.

Beatty, G. L., P. J. O'Dwyer, J. Clark, J. G. Shi, K. J. Bowman, P. A. Scherle, R. C. Newton, R. Schaub, J. Maleski, L. Leopold, and T. F. Gajewski. 2017. First-in-human Phase I study of the oral inhibitor of indoleamine 2,3-dioxygenase-1 epacadostat (INCB024360) in patients with advanced solid malignancies. *Clinical Cancer Research* 23(13):3269–3276.

Ben-David, U., and A. Amon. 2020. Context is everything: Aneuploidy in cancer. *Nature Reviews Genetics* 21(1):44–62.

Bensch, F., E. L. van der Veen, M. N. Lub-de Hooge, A. Jorritsma-Smit, R. Boellaard, I. C. Kok, S. F. Oosting, C. P. Schröder, T. J. N. Hiltermann, A. J. van der Wekken, H. J. M. Groen, T. C. Kwee, S. G. Elias, J. A. Gietema, S. S. Bohorquez, A. de Crespigny, S. P. Williams, C. Mancao, A. H. Brouwers, B. M. Fine, and E. G. E. de Vries. 2018. 89Zr-atezolizumab imaging as a non-invasive approach to assess clinical response to PD-L1 blockade in cancer. *Nature Medicine* 24(12):1852–1858.

Blumenthal, G. M., M. R. Theoret, and R. Pazdur. 2017. Treatment beyond progression with immune checkpoint inhibitors—known unknowns. *JAMA Oncology* 3(11):1473–1474.

Brown, C. C., H. Gudjonson, Y. Pritykin, D. Deep, V. P. Lavallée, A. Mendoza, R. Fromme, L. Mazutis, C. Ariyan, C. Leslie, D. Pe'er, and A. Y. Rudensky. 2019. Transcriptional basis of mouse and human dendritic cell heterogeneity. *Cell* 179(4):846–863.e24.

Burnell, S. E. A., L. Capitani, B. J. MacLachlan, G. H. Mason, A. M. Gallimore, and A. Godkin. 2021. Seven mysteries of LAG-3: A multi-faceted immune receptor of increasing complexity. *Immunotherapy Advances* 2(1):ltab025.

Buyse, M., D. J. Sargent, A. Grothey, A. Matheson, and A. de Gramont. 2010. Biomarkers and surrogate end points—the challenge of statistical validation. *Nature Reviews Clinical Oncology* 7(6):309–317.

Buzzatti, G., C. Dellepiane, and L. Del Mastro. 2020. New emerging targets in cancer immunotherapy: The role of GITR. *ESMO Open* 4(Suppl 3):e000738.

Cathcart-Rake, E. J., L. R. Sangaralingham, H. J. Henk, N. D. Shah, I. B. Riaz, and A. S. Mansfield. 2020. A population-based study of immunotherapy-related toxicities in lung cancer. *Clinical Lung Cancer* 21(5):421–427.e2.

Chan, J. M., Á. Quintanal-Villalonga, V. R. Gao, Y. Xie, V. Allaj, O. Chaudhary, I. Masilionis, J. Egger, A. Chow, T. Walle, M. Mattar, D. V. K. Yarlagadda, J. L. Wang, F. Uddin, M. Offin, M. Ciampricotti, B. Qeriqi, A. Bahr, E. de Stanchina, U. K. Bhanot, W. V. Lai, M. J. Bott, D. R. Jones, A. Ruiz, M. K. Baine, Y. Li, N. Rekhtman, J. T. Poirier, T. Nawy, T. Sen, L. Mazutis, T. J. Hollmann, D. Pe'er, and C. M. Rudin. 2021. Signatures of plasticity, metastasis, and immunosuppression in an atlas of human small cell lung cancer. *Cancer Cell* 39(11):1479–1496.e18.

Chang, E., L. Pelosof, S. Lemery, Y. Gong, K. B. Goldberg, A. T. Farrell, P. Keegan, J. Veeraraghavan, G. Wei, G. M. Blumenthal, L. Amiri-Kordestani, H. Singh, L. Fashoyin-Aje, N. Gormley, P. G. Kluetz, R. Pazdur, J. A. Beaver, and M. R. Theoret. 2021. Systematic review of PD-1/PD-l1 inhibitors in oncology: From personalized medicine to public health. *Oncologist* 26(10):e1786–e1799.

Chapman, P. B., L. H. Einhorn, M. L. Meyers, S. Saxman, A. N. Destro, K. S. Panageas, C. B. Begg, S. S. Agarwala, L. M. Schuchter, M. S. Ernstoff, A. N. Houghton, and J. M. Kirkwood. 1999. Phase III multicenter randomized trial of the Dartmouth regimen versus dacarbazine in patients with metastatic melanoma. *Journal of Clinical Oncology* 17(9):2745–2751.

Chen, D. S., and I. Mellman. 2013. Oncology meets immunology: The cancer-immunity cycle. *Immunity* 39(1):1–10.

Chen, G. M., C. Chen, R. K. Das, P. Gao, C. H. Chen, S. Bandyopadhyay, Y. Y. Ding, Y. Uzun, W. Yu, Q. Zhu, R. M. Myers, S. A. Grupp, D. M. Barrett, and K. Tan. 2021. Integrative bulk and single-cell profiling of premanufacture T-cell populations reveals factors mediating long-term persistence of CAR T-cell therapy. *Cancer Discovery* 11(9):2186–2199.

Chen, K. H., A. N. Boettiger, J. R. Moffitt, S. Wang, and X. Zhuang. 2015. RNA imaging. Spatially resolved, highly multiplexed RNA profiling in single cells. *Science* 348(6233):aaa6090.

Chen, P. L., W. Roh, A. Reuben, Z. A. Cooper, C. N. Spencer, P. A. Prieto, J. P. Miller, R. L. Bassett, V. Gopalakrishnan, K. Wani, M. P. De Macedo, J. L. Austin-Breneman, H. Jiang, Q. Chang, S. M. Reddy, W. S. Chen, M. T. Tetzlaff, R. J. Broaddus, M. A. Davies, J. E. Gershenwald, L. Haydu, A. J. Lazar, S. P. Patel, P. Hwu, W. J. Hwu, A. Diab, I. C. Glitza, S. E. Woodman, L. M. Vence, I. I. Wistuba, R. N. Amaria, L. N. Kwong, V. Prieto, R. E. Davis, W. Ma, W. W. Overwijk, A. H. Sharpe, J. Hu, P. A. Futreal, J. Blando, P. Sharma, J. P. Allison, L. Chin, and J. A. Wargo. 2016. Analysis of immune signatures in longitudinal tumor samples yields insight into biomarkers of response and mechanisms of resistance to immune checkpoint blockade. *Cancer Discovery* 6(8):827–837.

Cheong, J. E., and L. Sun. 2018. Targeting the IDO1/TDO2-KYN-AhR pathway for cancer immunotherapy: Challenges and opportunities. *Trends in Pharmacological Sciences* 39(3):307–325.

Chi, Y., J. Remsik, V. Kiseliovas, C. Derderian, U. Sener, M. Alghader, F. Saadeh, K. Nikishina, T. Bale, C. Iacobuzio-Donahue, T. Thomas, D. Pe'er, L. Mazutis, and A. Boire. 2020. Cancer cells deploy lipocalin-2 to collect limiting iron in leptomeningeal metastasis. *Science* 369(6501):276–282.

Choi, Y., Y. Shi, C. L. Haymaker, A. Naing, G. Ciliberto, and J. Hajjar. 2020. T-cell agonists in cancer immunotherapy. *Journal for Immunotherapy of Cancer* 8(2).

Chu, T., J. Berner, and D. Zehn. 2020. Two parallel worlds of memory T cells. *Nature Immunology* 21(12):1484–1485.

Cieri, N., B. Camisa, F. Cocchiarella, M. Forcato, G. Oliveira, E. Provasi, A. Bondanza, C. Bordignon, J. Peccatori, F. Ciceri, M. T. Lupo-Stanghellini, F. Mavilio, A. Mondino, S. Bicciato, A. Recchia, and C. Bonini. 2013. IL-7 and IL-15 instruct the generation of human memory stem T cells from naive precursors. *Blood* 121(4):573–584.

Cohen, A. D., D. A. Schaer, C. Liu, Y. Li, D. Hirschhorn-Cymmerman, S. C. Kim, A. Diab, G. Rizzuto, F. Duan, M. A. Perales, T. Merghoub, A. N. Houghton, and J. D. Wolchok. 2010. Agonist anti-GITR monoclonal antibody induces melanoma tumor immunity in mice by altering regulatory T cell stability and intra-tumor accumulation. *PLOS One* 5(5):e10436.

Comandè, G., and G. Schneider. 2018. Regulatory challenges of data mining practices: The case of the never-ending lifecycles of "health data." *European Journal of Health Law* 25:284–307.

Cortazar, P., and C. E. Geyer, Jr. 2015. Pathological complete response in neoadjuvant treatment of breast cancer. *Annals of Surgical Oncology* 22(5):1441–1446.

Cortazar, P., L. Zhang, M. Untch, K. Mehta, J. P. Costantino, N. Wolmark, H. Bonnefoi, D. Cameron, L. Gianni, P. Valagussa, S. M. Swain, T. Prowell, S. Loibl, D. L. Wickerham, J. Bogaerts, J. Baselga, C. Perou, G. Blumenthal, J. Blohmer, E. P. Mamounas, J. Bergh, V. Semiglazov, R. Justice, H. Eidtmann, S. Paik, M. Piccart, R. Sridhara, P. A. Fasching, L. Slaets, S. Tang, B. Gerber, C. E. Geyer, Jr., R. Pazdur, N. Ditsch, P. Rastogi, W. Eiermann, and G. von Minckwitz. 2014. Pathological complete response and long-term clinical benefit in breast cancer: The CTNeoBC pooled analysis. *Lancet* 384(9938):164–172.

D'Angelo, S. P., L. Melchiori, M. S. Merchant, D. Bernstein, J. Glod, R. Kaplan, S. Grupp, W. D. Tap, K. Chagin, G. K. Binder, S. Basu, D. E. Lowther, R. Wang, N. Bath, A. Tipping, G. Betts, I. Ramachandran, J. M. Navenot, H. Zhang, D. K. Wells, E. Van Winkle, G. Kari, T. Trivedi, T. Holdich, L. Pandite, R. Amado, and C. L. Mackall. 2018. Antitumor activity associated with prolonged persistence of adoptively transferred NY-ESO-1 c259T cells in synovial sarcoma. *Cancer Discovery* 8(8):944–957.

Davar, D., R. Zappasodi, H. Wang, G. S. Naik, T. Sato, T. Bauer, D. Bajor, O. Rixe, W. Newman, J. Qi, A. Holland, P. Wong, L. Sifferlen, D. Piper, C. A. Sirard, T. Merghoub, J. D. Wolchok, and J. J. Luke. 2022. Phase IB study of GITR agonist antibody TRX518 singly and in combination with gemcitabine, pembrolizumab, or nivolumab in patients with advanced solid tumors. *Clinical Cancer Research* 28(18):3990–4002.

Davis, E. J., J. Martin-Liberal, R. Kristeleit, D. C. Cho, S. P. Blagden, D. Berthold, D. B. Cardin, M. Vieito, R. E. Miller, P. H. Dass, A. Orcurto, K. Spencer, J. E. Janik, J. Clark, T. Condamine, J. Pulini, X. Chen, and J. M. Mehnert. 2022. First-in-human Phase I/II, open-label study of the anti-OX40 agonist INCAGN01949 in patients with advanced solid tumors. *The Journal for ImmunoTherapy of Cancer* 10(10):e004235.

Davis-Marcisak, E. F., A. Deshpande, G. L. Stein-O'Brien, W. J. Ho, D. Laheru, E. M. Jaffee, E. J. Fertig, and L. T. Kagohara. 2021. From bench to bedside: Single-cell analysis for cancer immunotherapy. *Cancer Cell* 39(8):1062–1080.

Day, D., A. M. Monjazeb, E. Sharon, S. P. Ivy, E. H. Rubin, G. L. Rosner, and M. O. Butler. 2017. From famine to feast: Developing early-phase combination immunotherapy trials wisely. *Clinical Cancer Research* 23(17):4980–4991.

Diab, A., H. J. Gogas, S. K. Sandhu, G. V. Long, P. A. Ascierto, J. Larkin, M. Sznol, F. A. Franke, T. Ciuleanu, E. Muñoz Couselo, A. Perfetti, C. Lebbe, F. Meier, B. Curti, C. Rojas, H. Yang, M. Zhou, S. Ravimohan, M. A. Tagliaferri, and N. Khushalani. 2022. 785O—PIVOT IO 001: First disclosure of efficacy and safety of bempegaldesleukin (BEMPEG) plus nivolumab (NIVO) vs. NIVO monotherapy in advanced melanoma (MEL). *Annals of Oncology* 33(suppl_7): S356–S409.

Dong, H., S. E. Strome, D. R. Salomao, H. Tamura, F. Hirano, D. B. Flies, P. C. Roche, J. Lu, G. Zhu, K. Tamada, V. A. Lennon, E. Celis, and L. Chen. 2002. Tumor-associated B7-H1 promotes T-cell apoptosis: A potential mechanism of immune evasion. *Nature Medicine* 8(8):793–800.

Esfahani, K., A. Elkrief, C. Calabrese, R. Lapointe, M. Hudson, B. Routy, W. H. Miller, Jr., and L. Calabrese. 2020. Moving towards personalized treatments of immune-related adverse events. *Nature Reviews Clinical Oncology* 17(8):504–515.

Farwell, M. D., R. F. Gamache, H. Babazada, M. D. Hellmann, J. J. Harding, R. Korn, A. Mascioni, W. Le, I. Wilson, M. S. Gordon, A. M. Wu, G. A. Ulaner, J. D. Wolchok, M. A. Postow, and N. Pandit-Taskar. 2022. CD8-targeted PET imaging of tumor-infiltrating T cells in patients with cancer: A Phase I first-in-humans study of 89Zr-Df-IAB22M2C, a radiolabeled anti-CD8 minibody. *Journal of Nuclear Medicine* 63(5):720–726.

FDA (U.S. Food and Drug Administration). 2013. Codevelopment of two or more new investigational drugs for use in combination. https://www.fda.gov/regulatory-information/search-fda-guidance-documents/codevelopment-two-or-more-new-investigational-drugs-use-combination (accessed January 11, 2023).

FDA. 2019. FDA warns about the risks associated with the investigational use of Venclexta in multiple myeloma [Press release]. https://www.fda.gov/drugs/drug-safety-and-availability/fda-warns-about-risks-associated-investigational-use-venclexta-multiple-myeloma (accessed December 20, 2022).

Foster, J. C., B. Freidlin, C. A. Kunos, and E. L. Korn. 2020. Single-arm Phase II trials of combination therapies: A review of the CTEP experience 2008–2017. *Journal of the National Cancer Institute* 112(2):128–135.

Frey, N. V., S. Gill, W. T. Hwang, S. M. Luger, M. E. Martin, S. R. McCurdy, A. W. Loren, K. W. Pratz, A. E. Perl, J. Barber-Rotenberg, A. Marshall, M. Ruella, S. F. Lacey, J. Fraietta, A. Fesnak, M. O'Brien, T. Schanne, J. L. Brogdon, B. Engels, B. L. Levine, C. H. June, D. L. Porter, and E. O. Hexner. 2021. CART22-65s co-administered with huCART19 in adult patients with relapsed or refractory ALL. *Blood* 138(Supplement 1):469.

Fröhlich, H., R. Balling, N. Beerenwinkel, O. Kohlbacher, S. Kumar, T. Lengauer, M. H. Maathuis, Y. Moreau, S. A. Murphy, T. M. Przytycka, M. Rebhan, H. Röst, A. Schuppert, M. Schwab, R. Spang, D. Stekhoven, J. Sun, A. Weber, D. Ziemek, and B. Zupan. 2018. From hype to reality: Data science enabling personalized medicine. *BMC Medicine* 16(1):150.

Ganahl, M., J. Beall, M. Hauru, A. G. M. Lewis, J. H. Yoo, Y. Zou, and G. Vidal. 2022. Density matrix renormalization group with Tensor Processing Units. *arXiv Condensed Matter*:2204.05693.

Gattinoni, L., E. Lugli, Y. Ji, Z. Pos, C. M. Paulos, M. F. Quigley, J. R. Almeida, E. Gostick, Z. Yu, C. Carpenito, E. Wang, D. C. Douek, D. A. Price, C. H. June, F. M. Marincola, M. Roederer, and N. P. Restifo. 2011. A human memory T cell subset with stem cell-like properties. *Nature Medicine* 17(10):1290–1297.

Gormley, N. J., A. T. Farrell, and R. Pazdur. 2017. Minimal residual disease as a potential surrogate end point—lingering questions. *JAMA Oncology* 3(1):18–20.

Guo, W., Y. Pang, L. Yao, L. Zhao, C. Fan, J. Ke, P. Guo, B. Hao, H. Fu, C. Xie, Q. Lin, H. Wu, L. Sun, and H. Chen. 2021. Imaging fibroblast activation protein in liver cancer: A single-center post hoc retrospective analysis to compare [68Ga]Ga-FAPI-04 PET/CT versus MRI and [18F]-FDG PET/CT. *European Journal of Nuclear Medicine and Molecular Imaging* 48(5):1604–1617.

Hamid, O., T. F. Gajewski, A. E. Frankel, T. M. Bauer, A. J. Olszanski, J. J. Luke, A. S. Balmanoukian, E. V. Schmidt, B. Sharkey, J. Maleski, M. J. Jones, and T. C. Gangadhar. 2017. Epacadostat plus pembrolizumab in patients with advanced melanoma: Phase 1 and 2 efficacy and safety results from ECHO-202/KEYNOTE-037. *Abstracts: Melanoma and Other Skin Tumours* 28(5):V428–V429.

Han, G., G. Yang, D. Hao, Y. Lu, K. Thein, B. S. Simpson, J. Chen, R. Sun, O. Alhalabi, R. Wang, M. Dang, E. Dai, S. Zhang, F. Nie, S. Zhao, C. Guo, A. Hamza, B. Czerniak, C. Cheng, A. Siefker-Radtke, K. Bhat, A. Futreal, G. Peng, J. Wargo, W. Peng, H. Kadara, J. Ajani, C. Swanton, K. Litchfield, J. R. Ahnert, J. Gao, and L. Wang. 2021. 9p21 loss confers a cold tumor immune microenvironment and primary resistance to immune checkpoint therapy. *Nature Communications* 12(1):5606.

Hariton, E., and J. J. Locascio. 2018. Randomised controlled trials—the gold standard for effectiveness research: Study design: Randomised controlled trials. *BJOG: An International Journal of Obstetrics & Gynaecology* 125(13):1716.

Hauru, M., A. Morningstar, J. Beall, M. Ganahl, A. Lewis, and G. Vidal. 2021. Simulation of quantum physics with Tensor Processing Units: Brute-force computation of ground states and time evolution. *arXiv Quantum Physics*:2111.10466.

Hirsch, F. R., A. McElhinny, D. Stanforth, J. Ranger-Moore, M. Jansson, K. Kulangara, W. Richardson, P. Towne, D. Hanks, B. Vennapusa, A. Mistry, R. Kalamegham, S. Averbuch, J. Novotny, E. Rubin, K. Emancipator, I. McCaffery, J. A. Williams, J. Walker, J. Longshore, M. S. Tsao, and K. M. Kerr. 2017. PD-L1 immunohistochemistry assays for lung cancer: Results from Phase 1 of the Blueprint PD-L1 IHC Assay Comparison Project. *The Journal of Thoracic Oncology* 12(2):208–222.

Huang, X., T. Tian, Y. Zhang, S. Zhou, P. Hu, and J. Zhang. 2021. Age-associated changes in adverse events arising from anti-PD-(L)1 therapy. *Frontiers in Oncology* 11:619385.

Huo, J. L., Y. T. Wang, W. J. Fu, N. Lu, and Z. S. Liu. 2022. The promising immune checkpoint LAG-3 in cancer immunotherapy: From basic research to clinical application. *Frontiers in Immunology* 13:956090.

Hurwitz, M. E., D. C. Cho, A. V. Balar, B. D. Curti, A. O. Siefker-Radtke, M. Sznol, H. M. Kluger, C. Bernatchez, C. Fanton, E. Iacucci, Y. Liu, T. Nguyen, W. Overwijk, J. Zalevsky, M. A. Tagliaferri, U. Hoch, and A. Diab. 2019. Baseline tumor-immune signatures associated with response to bempegaldesleukin (NKTR-214) and nivolumab. *Journal of Clinical Oncology* 37(15_suppl):2623.

Ibrahim, O., and J. O'Sullivan. 2020. Iron chelators in cancer therapy. *Biometals* 33(4–5):201–215.

Idera Pharmaceuticals. 2021. Idera Pharmaceuticals announces results from Illuminate-301 trial of tilsotolimod + ipilimumab in anti-PD-1 refractory advanced melanoma [Press release]. https://ir.iderapharma.com/news-releases/news-release-details/idera-pharmaceuticals-announces-results-illuminate-301-trial (accessed December 12, 2022).

Jauw, Y. W., J. M. Zijlstra, D. de Jong, D. J. Vugts, S. Zweegman, O. S. Hoekstra, G. A. van Dongen, and M. C. Huisman. 2017. Performance of 89Zr-labeled-rituximab-PET as an imaging biomarker to assess CD20 targeting: A pilot study in patients with relapsed/refractory diffuse large B cell lymphoma. *PLOS One* 12(1):e0169828.

Jenkins, R. W., A. R. Aref, P. H. Lizotte, E. Ivanova, S. Stinson, C. W. Zhou, M. Bowden, J. Deng, H. Liu, D. Miao, M. X. He, W. Walker, G. Zhang, T. Tian, C. Cheng, Z. Wei, S. Palakurthi, M. Bittinger, H. Vitzthum, J. W. Kim, A. Merlino, M. Quinn, C. Venkataramani, J. A. Kaplan, A. Portell, P. C. Gokhale, B. Phillips, A. Smart, A. Rotem, R. E. Jones, L. Keogh, M. Anguiano, L. Stapleton, Z. Jia, M. Barzily-Rokni, I. Cañadas, T. C. Thai, M. R. Hammond, R. Vlahos, E. S. Wang, H. Zhang, S. Li, G. J. Hanna, W. Huang, M. P. Hoang, A. Piris, J. P. Eliane, A. O. Stemmer-Rachamimov, L. Cameron, M. J. Su, P. Shah, B. Izar, M. Thakuria, N. R. LeBoeuf, G. Rabinowits, V. Gunda, S. Parangi, J. M. Cleary, B. C. Miller, S. Kitajima, R. Thummalapalli, B. Miao, T. U. Barbie, V. Sivathanu, J. Wong, W. G. Richards, R. Bueno, C. H. Yoon, J. Miret, M. Herlyn, L. A. Garraway, E. M. Van Allen, G. J. Freeman, P. T. Kirschmeier, J. H. Lorch, P. A. Ott, F. S. Hodi, K. T. Flaherty, R. D. Kamm, G. M. Boland, K. K. Wong, D. Dornan, C. P. Paweletz, and D. A. Barbie. 2018. Ex vivo profiling of PD-1 blockade using organotypic tumor spheroids. *Cancer Discovery* 8(2):196–215.

Jhunjhunwala, S., C. Hammer, and L. Delamarre. 2021. Antigen presentation in cancer: Insights into tumour immunogenicity and immune evasion. *Nature Reviews Cancer* 21(5):298–312.

Jia, W., Q. Gao, A. Han, H. Zhu, and J. Yu. 2019. The potential mechanism, recognition and clinical significance of tumor pseudoprogression after immunotherapy. *Cancer Biology & Medicine* 16(4):655–670.

Jonas, O., H. M. Landry, J. E. Fuller, J. T. Santini, Jr., J. Baselga, R. I. Tepper, M. J. Cima, and R. Langer. 2015. An implantable microdevice to perform high-throughput in vivo drug sensitivity testing in tumors. *Science Translational Medicine* 7(284):284ra257.

Kluger, H. M., H. A. Tawbi, M. L. Ascierto, M. Bowden, M. K. Callahan, E. Cha, X. Chen, C. G. Drake, D. M. Feltquate, R. L. Ferris, J. L. Gulley, S. Gupta, R. W. Humphrey, T. M. LaVallee, D. T. Le, V. M. Hubbard-Lucey, V. A. Papadimitrakopoulou, M. A. Postow, E. H. Rubin, E. Sharon, J. M. Taube, S. L. Topalian, R. Zappasodi, M. Sznol, and R. J. Sullivan. 2020. Defining tumor resistance to PD-1 pathway blockade: Recommendations from the first meeting of the SITC Immunotherapy Resistance Taskforce. *The Journal for ImmunoTherapy of Cancer* 8(1):e000398.

Knouse, K. A., T. Davoli, S. J. Elledge, and A. Amon. 2017. Aneuploidy in cancer: Seq-ing answers to old questions. *Annual Review of Cancer Biology* 1:335–354.

Kratochwil, C., P. Flechsig, T. Lindner, L. Abderrahim, A. Altmann, W. Mier, S. Adeberg, H. Rathke, M. Röhrich, H. Winter, P. K. Plinkert, F. Marme, M. Lang, H. U. Kauczor, D. Jäger, J. Debus, U. Haberkorn, and F. L. Giesel. 2019. 68Ga-FAPI PET/CT: Tracer uptake in 28 different kinds of cancer. *The Journal of Nuclear Medicine* 60(6):801–805.

Kunes, R. Z., T. Walle, M. Land, T. Nawy, and D. Pe'er. 2023. Supervised discovery of interpretable gene programs from single-cell data. *Nature Biotechnology*. https://doi.org/10.1038/s41587-023-01940-3.

Labadie, B. W., R. Bao, and J. J. Luke. 2019. Reimagining IDO pathway inhibition in cancer immunotherapy via downstream focus on the tryptophan-kynurenine-aryl hydrocarbon axis. *Clinical Cancer Research* 25(5):1462–1471.

Lancet Oncology. 2018. Minimalism in oncology [Editorial]. *The Lancet Oncology* 19(5):579.

Landgren, O., S. Devlin, M. Boulad, and S. Mailankody. 2016. Role of MRD status in relation to clinical outcomes in newly diagnosed multiple myeloma patients: A meta-analysis. *Bone Marrow Transplantation* 51(12):1565–1568.

Lapteva, L., T. Purohit-Sheth, M. Serabian, and R. K. Puri. 2020. Clinical development of gene therapies: The first three decades and counting. *Molecular Therapy. Methods & Clinical Development* 19:387–397.

Larkin, J., V. Chiarion-Sileni, R. Gonzalez, J. J. Grob, C. L. Cowey, C. D. Lao, D. Schadendorf, R. Dummer, M. Smylie, P. Rutkowski, P. F. Ferrucci, A. Hill, J. Wagstaff, M. S. Carlino, J. B. Haanen, M. Maio, I. Marquez-Rodas, G. A. McArthur, P. A. Ascierto, G. V. Long, M. K. Callahan, M. A. Postow, K. Grossmann, M. Sznol, B. Dreno, L. Bastholt, A. Yang, L. M. Rollin, C. Horak, F. S. Hodi, and J. D. Wolchok. 2015. Combined nivolumab and ipilimumab or monotherapy in untreated melanoma. *New England Journal of Medicine* 373(1):23–34.

Larkin, J., M. Oya, M. Martignoni, F. Thistlethwaite, P. Nathan, M. C. Ornstein, T. Powles, K. E. Beckermann, A. V. Balar, D. McDermott, S. Gupta, G. K. Philips, M. S. Gordon, H. Uemura, Y. Tomita, J. Wang, E. Michelon, A. di Pietro, and T. K. Choueiri. 2022. Avelumab plus axitinib as first-line therapy for advanced renal cell carcinoma: Long-term results from the JAVELIN renal 100 Phase Ib trial. *Oncologist* (28):oyac243.

Laughney, A. M., J. Hu, N. R. Campbell, S. F. Bakhoum, M. Setty, V. P. Lavallée, Y. Xie, I. Masilionis, A. J. Carr, S. Kottapalli, V. Allaj, M. Mattar, N. Rekhtman, J. B. Xavier, L. Mazutis, J. T. Poirier, C. M. Rudin, D. Pe'er, and J. Massagué. 2020. Regenerative lineages and immune-mediated pruning in lung cancer metastasis. *Nature Medicine* 26(2):259–269.

Le, D. T., J. N. Uram, H. Wang, B. R. Bartlett, H. Kemberling, A. D. Eyring, A. D. Skora, B. S. Luber, N. S. Azad, D. Laheru, B. Biedrzycki, R. C. Donehower, A. Zaheer, G. A. Fisher, T. S. Crocenzi, J. J. Lee, S. M. Duffy, R. M. Goldberg, A. de la Chapelle, M. Koshiji, F. Bhaijee, T. Huebner, R. H. Hruban, L. D. Wood, N. Cuka, D. M. Pardoll, N. Papadopoulos, K. W. Kinzler, S. Zhou, T. C. Cornish, J. M. Taube, R. A. Anders, J. R. Eshleman, B. Vogelstein, and L. A. Diaz, Jr. 2015. PD-1 blockade in tumors with mismatch-repair deficiency. *The New England Journal of Medicine* 372(26):2509–2520.

Leach, D. R., M. F. Krummel, and J. P. Allison. 1996. Enhancement of antitumor immunity by CTLA-4 blockade. *Science* 271(5256):1734–1736.

Lemery, S., P. Keegan, and R. Pazdur. 2017. First FDA approval agnostic of cancer site - when a biomarker defines the indication. *New England Journal of Medicine* 377(15):1409-1412.

Levin, N., B. C. Paria, N. R. Vale, R. Yossef, F. J. Lowery, M. R. Parkhurst, Z. Yu, M. Florentin, G. Cafri, J. J. Gartner, M. L. Shindorf, L. T. Ngo, S. Ray, S. P. Kim, A. R. Copeland, P. F. Robbins, and S. A. Rosenberg. 2021. Identification and validation of T-cell receptors targeting RAS hotspot mutations in human cancers for use in cell-based immunotherapy. *Clinical Cancer Research* 27(18):5084–5095.

Linch, S. N., M. J. McNamara, and W. L. Redmond. 2015. Ox40 agonists and combination immunotherapy: Putting the pedal to the metal. *Frontiers in Oncology* 5:34.

Lipson, E. J., W. H. Sharfman, C. G. Drake, I. Wollner, J. M. Taube, R. A. Anders, H. Xu, S. Yao, A. Pons, L. Chen, D. M. Pardoll, J. R. Brahmer, and S. L. Topalian. 2013. Durable cancer regression off-treatment and effective reinduction therapy with an anti-PD-1 antibody. *Clinical Cancer Research* 19(2):462–468.

Lipson, E. J., H. A. Tawbi, D. Schadendorf, P. A. Ascierto, L. Matamala, E. Castillo Gutiérrez, P. Rutkowski, H. Gogas, C. D. Lao, J. J. de Menezes, S. Dalle, A. M. Arance, J. J. Grob, S. Srivastava, M. Abaskharoun, K. L. Simonsen, B. Li, G. V. Long, and F. S. Hodi. 2021. Relatlimab (RELA) plus nivolumab (NIVO) versus NIVO in first-line advanced melanoma: Primary Phase III results from RELATIVITY-047 (CA224-047). *Journal of Clinical Oncology* 39(15_suppl):9503.

Long, G. V., R. Dummer, O. Hamid, T. F. Gajewski, C. Caglevic, S. Dalle, A. Arance, M. S. Carlino, J. J. Grob, T. M. Kim, L. Demidov, C. Robert, J. Larkin, J. R. Anderson, J. Maleski, M. Jones, S. J. Diede, and T. C. Mitchell. 2019. Epacadostat plus pembrolizumab versus placebo plus pembrolizumab in patients with unresectable or metastatic melanoma (ECHO-301/KEYNOTE-252): A Phase 3, randomised, double-blind study. *Lancet Oncology* 20(8):1083–1097.

Luke, J. J., J. Tabernero, A. Joshua, J. Desai, A. I. Varga, V. Moreno, C. A. Gomez-Roca, B. Markman, F. G. De Braud, S. Pravin Patel, M. S. Carlino, L. L. Siu, G. Curigliano, Z. Liu, Y. Ishii, M. Wind-Rotolo, P. A. Basciano, A. Azrilevich, and K. A. Gelmon. 2019. BMS-986205, an indoleamine 2, 3-dioxygenase 1 inhibitor (IDO1i), in combination with nivolumab (NIVO): Updated safety across all tumor cohorts and efficacy in advanced bladder cancer (advBC). *Journal of Clinical Oncology* 37(7_suppl):358.

Makkouk, A., and G. J. Weiner. 2015. Cancer immunotherapy and breaking immune tolerance: New approaches to an old challenge. *Cancer Research* 75(1):5–10.

Malik, S. M., R. Pazdur, J. S. Abrams, M. A. Socinski, W. T. Sause, D. H. Harpole, Jr., J. J. Welch, E. L. Korn, C. D. Ullmann, and F. R. Hirsch. 2014. Consensus report of a joint NCI Thoracic Malignancies Steering Committee: FDA workshop on strategies for integrating biomarkers into clinical development of new therapies for lung cancer leading to the inception of "master protocols" in lung cancer. *Journal of Thoracic Oncology* 9(10):1443–1448.

Marofi, F., R. Motavalli, V. A. Safonov, L. Thangavelu, A. V. Yumashev, M. Alexander, N. Shomali, M. S. Chartrand, Y. Pathak, M. Jarahian, S. Izadi, A. Hassanzadeh, N. Shirafkan, S. Tahmasebi, and F. M. Khiavi. 2021. CAR T cells in solid tumors: Challenges and opportunities. *Stem Cell Research and Therapy* 12(1):81.

Mayoux, M., A. Roller, V. Pulko, S. Sammicheli, S. Chen, E. Sum, C. Jost, M. F. Fransen, R. B. Buser, M. Kowanetz, K. Rommel, I. Matos, S. Colombetti, A. Belousov, V. Karanikas, F. Ossendorp, P. S. Hegde, D. S. Chen, P. Umana, M. Perro, C. Klein, and W. Xu. 2020. Dendritic cells dictate responses to PD-L1 blockade cancer immunotherapy. *Science Translational Medicine* 12(534):eaav7431.

McGovern, K., A. C. Castro, J. Cavanaugh, S. Coma, M. Walsh, J. Tchaicha, S. Syed, P. Natarajan, M. Manfredi, X. M. Zhang, and J. Ecsedy. 2022. Discovery and characterization of a novel aryl hydrocarbon receptor inhibitor, IK-175, and its inhibitory activity on tumor immune suppression. *Molecular Cancer Therapeutics* 21(8):1261–1272.

Messenheimer, D. J., S. M. Jensen, M. E. Afentoulis, K. W. Wegmann, Z. Feng, D. J. Friedman, M. J. Gough, W. J. Urba, and B. A. Fox. 2017. Timing of PD-1 blockade is critical to effective combination immunotherapy with anti-OX40. *Clinical Cancer Research* 23(20):6165–6177.

Mitchell, T. C., O. Hamid, D. C. Smith, T. M. Bauer, J. S. Wasser, A. J. Olszanski, J. J. Luke, A. S. Balmanoukian, E. V. Schmidt, Y. Zhao, X. Gong, J. Maleski, L. Leopold, and T. F. Gajewski. 2018. Epacadostat plus pembrolizumab in patients with advanced solid tumors: Phase I results from a multicenter, open-label Phase I/II trial (ECHO-202/ KEYNOTE-037). *Journal of Clinical Oncology* 36(32):3223–3230.

Mohanty, S., M. Aghighi, K. Yerneni, J. L. Theruvath, and H. E. Daldrup-Link. 2019a. Improving the efficacy of osteosarcoma therapy: Combining drugs that turn cancer cell "don't eat me" signals off and "eat me" signals on. *Molecular Oncology* 10:18780261.

Mohanty, S., K. Yerneni, J. L. Theruvath, C. M. Graef, H. Nejadnik, O. Lenkov, L. Pisani, J. Rosenberg, S. Mitra, A. Sweet Cordero, S. Cheshier, and H. E. Daldrup-Link. 2019b. Nanoparticle enhanced MRI can monitor macrophage response to CD47 mAb immunotherapy in osteosarcoma. *Cell Death and Disease* 10:36.

Muik, A., E. Garralda, I. Altintas, F. Gieseke, R. Geva, E. Ben-Ami, C. Maurice-Dror, E. Calvo, P. M. LoRusso, G. Alonso, M. E. Rodriguez-Ruiz, K. B. Schoedel, J. M. Blum, B. Sänger, T. W. Salcedo, S. M. Burm, E. Stanganello, D. Verzijl, F. Vascotto, A. Sette, J. Quinkhardt, T. S. Plantinga, A. Toker, E. N. van den Brink, M. Fereshteh, M. Diken, D. Satijn, S. Kreiter, E. C. W. Breij, G. Bajaj, E. Lagkadinou, K. Sasser, Ö. Türeci, U. Forssmann, T. Ahmadi, U. Şahin, M. Jure-Kunkel, and I. Melero. 2022. Preclinical characterization and Phase I trial results of a bispecific antibody targeting PD-L1 and 4-1BB (GEN1046) in patients with advanced refractory solid tumors. *Cancer Discovery* 12(5):1248–1265.

Mulkey, F., M. R. Theoret, P. Keegan, R. Pazdur, and R. Sridhara. 2020. Comparison of iRECIST versus RECIST V.1.1 in patients treated with an anti-PD-1 or PD-L1 antibody: Pooled FDA analysis. *Journal for ImmunoTherapy of Cancer* 8(1):e000146.

Munshi, N. C., H. Avet-Loiseau, A. C. Rawstron, R. G. Owen, J. A. Child, A. Thakurta, P. Sherrington, M. K. Samur, A. Georgieva, K. C. Anderson, and W. M. Gregory. 2017. Association of minimal residual disease with superior survival outcomes in patients with multiple myeloma: A meta-analysis. *JAMA Oncology* 3(1):28–35.

Murray, I. A., A. D. Patterson, and G. H. Perdew. 2014. Aryl hydrocarbon receptor ligands in cancer: Friend and foe. *Nature Reviews Cancer* 14(12):801–814.

Nadkarni, P. M., L. Ohno-Machado, and W. W. Chapman. 2011. Natural language processing: An introduction. *Journal of the American Medical Informatics Association* 18(5):544–551.

NASEM (National Academies of Sciences, Engineering, and Medicine). 2016. *Policy issues in the clinical development and use of immunotherapy for cancer treatment: Proceedings of a workshop.* Washington, DC: The National Academies Press.

NASEM. 2019. *Advancing progress in the development of combination cancer therapies with immune checkpoint inhibitors: Proceedings of a workshop.* Washington, DC: The National Academies Press.

National Library of Medicine. 2021. An investigational immuno-therapy study of BMS-986205 combined with nivolumab, compared to nivolumab by itself, in patients with advanced melanoma. https://clinicaltrials.gov/ct2/show/NCT03329846 (accessed May 11, 2023).

NCI (National Cancer Institute). 2023. NCI dictionary of cancer terms: Immune system modulator. https://www.cancer.gov/publications/dictionaries/cancer-terms/def/ immune-system-modulator (accessed March 21, 2023).

Nebert, D. W., and G. Zhang. 2019. Pharmacogenomics. In *Emery and Rimoin's Principles and Practice of Medical Genetics and Genomics*, 445–486.

Oh, S. A., D. C. Wu, J. Cheung, A. Navarro, H. Xiong, R. Cubas, K. Totpal, H. Chiu, Y. Wu, L. Comps-Agrar, A. M. Leader, M. Merad, M. Roose-Germa, S. Warming, M. Yan, J. M. Kim, S. Rutz, and I. Mellman. 2020. PD-L1 expression by dendritic cells is a key regulator of T-cell immunity in cancer. *Nature Cancer* 1(7):681–691.

Osterman, T. J., M. Terry, and R. S. Miller. 2020. Improving cancer data interoperability: The promise of the Minimal Common Oncology Data Elements (mCODE) initiative. *JCO Clinical Cancer Informatics* 4:993–1001.

Pandit-Taskar, N., M. A. Postow, M. D. Hellmann, J. J. Harding, C. A. Barker, J. A. O'Donoghue, M. Ziolkowska, S. Ruan, S. K. Lyashchenko, F. Tsai, M. Farwell, T. C. Mitchell, R. Korn, W. Le, J. S. Lewis, W. A. Weber, D. Behera, I. Wilson, M. Gordon, A. M. Wu, and J. D. Wolchok. 2022. First-in-humans imaging with 89Zr-Df-IAB22M2C anti-CD8 minibody in patients with solid malignancies: Preliminary pharmacokinetics, biodistribution, and lesion targeting. *Journal of Nuclear Medicine* 61(4):512–519.

Park, H. J., K. W. Kim, J. Pyo, C. H. Suh, S. Yoon, H. Hatabu, and M. Nishino. 2020. Incidence of pseudoprogression during immune checkpoint inhibitor therapy for solid tumors: A systematic review and meta-analysis. *Radiology* 297(1):87–96.

Paul, W. E., ed. 2003. *Fundamental Immunology*. 5th edition. Philadelphia: Lippincott Williams & Wilkins.

Pederson, R., J. Kozlowski, R. Song, J. Beall, M. Ganahl, M. Hauru, A. G. M. Lewis, Y. Yao, S. B. Mallick, V. Blum, and G. Vidal. 2022. Large scale quantum chemistry with Tensor Processing Units. *Journal of Chemical Theory and Computation* 19(1):25–32. https://doi.org/10.48550/arXiv.2202.01255.

Pereira, B. A., C. Vennin, M. Papanicolaou, C. R. Chambers, D. Herrmann, J. P. Morton, T. R. Cox, and P. Timpson. 2019. CAF subpopulations: A new reservoir of stromal targets in pancreatic cancer. *Trends in Cancer* 5(11):724–741.

Postow, M. A., M. K. Callahan, and J. D. Wolchok. 2015. Immune checkpoint blockade in cancer therapy. *Journal of Clinical Oncology* 33(17):1974–1982.

Powles, T., S. H. Park, E. Voog, C. Caserta, B. Pérez-Valderrama, H. Gurney, Y. Loriot, S. S. Sridhar, N. Tsuchiya, C. N. Sternberg, J. Bellmunt, J. B. Aragon-Ching, D. P. Petrylak, A. Blake-Haskins, R. J. Laliberte, J. Wang, N. M. Costa, and P. Grivas. 2023. Avelumab first-line (1L) maintenance for advanced urothelial carcinoma (UC): Long-term follow-up results from the JAVELIN Bladder 100 trial. *Journal of Clinical Oncology* 41(19):3486-3492.

Prentice, R. L. 1989. Surrogate endpoints in clinical trials: Definition and operational criteria. *Statistics in Medicine* 8(4):431–440.

Propper, D. J., and F. R. Balkwill. 2022. Harnessing cytokines and chemokines for cancer therapy. *Nature Reviews Clinical Oncology* 19:237–253.

Radtke, A. J., E. Kandov, B. Lowekamp, E. Speranza, C. J. Chu, A. Gola, N. Thakur, R. Shih, L. Yao, Z. R. Yaniv, R. T. Beuschel, J. Kabat, J. Croteau, J. Davis, J. M. Hernandez, and R. N. Germain. 2020. Ibex: A versatile multiplex optical imaging approach for deep phenotyping and spatial analysis of cells in complex tissues. *Proceedings of the National Academy of Sciences* 117(52):33455–33465.

Reckamp, K. L., M. W. Redman, K. H. Dragnev, K. Minichiello, L. C. Villaruz, B. Faller, T. Al Baghdadi, S. Hines, L. Everhart, L. Highleyman, V. Papadimitrakopoulou, J. W. Neal, S. N. Waqar, J. D. Patel, J. E. Gray, D. R. Gandara, K. Kelly, and R. S. Herbst. 2022. Phase II randomized study of ramucirumab and pembrolizumab versus standard of care in advanced non-small-cell lung cancer previously treated with immunotherapy-Lung-MAP S1800A. *Journal of Clinical Oncology* 40(21):2295–2306.

Reinfeld, B. I., M. Z. Madden, M. M. Wolf, A. Chytil, J. E. Bader, A. R. Patterson, A. Sugiura, A. S. Cohen, A. Ali, B. T. Do, A. Muir, C. A. Lewis, R. A. Hongo, K. L. Young, R. E. Brown, V. M. Todd, T. Huffstater, A. Abraham, R. T. O'Neil, M. H. Wilson, F. Xin, N. M. Tantawy, W. D. Merryman, R. W. Johnson, C. S. Williams, E. F. Mason, F. M. Mason, K. E. Beckermann, M. G. Vander Heiden, H. C. Manning, J. C. Rathmell, and W. K. Rathmell. 2021. Cell-programmed nutrient partitioning in the tumour microenvironment. *Nature* 593(7858):282–288.

Ruffo, E., R. C. Wu, T. C. Bruno, C. J. Workman, and D. A. A. Vignali. 2019. Lymphocyte-activation gene 3 (LAG3): The next immune checkpoint receptor. *Seminars in Immunology* 42:101305.

Sade-Feldman, M., K. Yizhak, S. L. Bjorgaard, J. P. Ray, C. G. de Boer, R. W. Jenkins, D. J. Lieb, J. H. Chen, D. T. Frederick, M. Barzily-Rokni, S. S. Freeman, A. Reuben, P. J. Hoover, A. C. Villani, E. Ivanova, A. Portell, P. H. Lizotte, A. R. Aref, J. P. Eliane, M. R. Hammond, H. Vitzthum, S. M. Blackmon, B. Li, V. Gopalakrishnan, S. M. Reddy, Z. A. Cooper, C. P. Paweletz, D. A. Barbie, A. Stemmer-Rachamimov, K. T. Flaherty, J. A. Wargo, G. M. Boland, R. J. Sullivan, G. Getz, and N. Hacohen. 2018. Defining T cell states associated with response to checkpoint immunotherapy in melanoma. *Cell* 175(4):998–1013.e20.

Sakhiya, J., D. Sakhiya, J. Kaklotar, B. Hirapara, M. Purohit, K. Bhalala, F. Daruwala, and N. Dudhatra. 2021. Intralesional agents in dermatology: Pros and cons. *Journal of Cutaneous Aesthetic Surgery* 14(3):285–295.

Sargent, D. J., and S. J. Mandrekar. 2013. Statistical issues in the validation of prognostic, predictive, and surrogate biomarkers. *Clinical Trials* 10(5):647–652.

Sargent, D. J., Q. Shi, S. De Bedout, C. Flowers, N. H. Fowler, T. Fu, A. Hagenbeek, M. Herold, E. Hoster, J. Huang, E. Kimby, M. Ladetto, F. Morschhauser, T. Nielsen, K. Takeshita, N. Valente, U. Vitolo, E. Zucca, G. A. Salles, and the FLASH (Follicular Lymphoma Analysis of Surrogacy Hypothesis) Group. 2015. Evaluation of complete response rate at 30 months (CR30) as a surrogate for progression-free survival (PFS) in first-line follicular lymphoma (FL) studies: Results from the prospectively specified Follicular Lymphoma Analysis of Surrogacy Hypothesis (FLASH) analysis with individual patient data (IPD) of 3,837 patients (pts). *Journal of Clinical Oncology* 33(15_suppl):8504.

Schadendorf, D., F. S. Hodi, C. Robert, J. S. Weber, K. Margolin, O. Hamid, D. Patt, T. T. Chen, D. M. Berman, and J. D. Wolchok. 2015. Pooled analysis of long-term survival data from Phase II and Phase III trials of ipilimumab in unresectable or metastatic melanoma. *Journal of Clinical Oncology* 33(17):1889–1894.

Schoenfeld, A. J., and M. D. Hellmann. 2020. Acquired resistance to immune checkpoint inhibitors. *Cancer Cell* 37(4):443–455.

Sehgal, K., A. Portell, E. V. Ivanova, P. H. Lizotte, N. R. Mahadevan, J. R. Greene, A. Vajdi, C. Gurjao, T. Teceno, L. J. Taus, T. C. Thai, S. Kitajima, D. Liu, T. Tani, M. Noureddine, C. J. Lau, P. T. Kirschmeier, D. Liu, M. Giannakis, R. W. Jenkins, P. C. Gokhale, S. Goldoni, M. Pinzon-Ortiz, W. D. Hastings, P. S. Hammerman, J. J. Miret, C. P. Paweletz, and D. A. Barbie. 2021. Dynamic single-cell RNA sequencing identifies immunotherapy persister cells following PD-1 blockade. *Journal of Clinical Investigation* 131(2):e135038.

Seliger, B., and C. Massa. 2021. Immune therapy resistance and immune escape of tumors. *Cancers* 13(3):551.

Shah, M., A. Rahman, M. R. Theoret, and R. Pazdur. 2021. The drug-dosing conundrum in oncology—When less is more. *New England Journal of Medicine* 385(16):1445–1447.

Sharma, P., S. Hu-Lieskovan, J. A. Wargo, and A. Ribas. 2017. Primary, adaptive, and acquired resistance to cancer immunotherapy. *Cell* 168(4):707–723.

Sharon, E., and J. C. Foster. 2023. Design of phase II oncology trials evaluating combinations of experimental agents. *JNCI: Journal of the National Cancer Institute* 115(6):613-618.

Shrimali, R. K., S. Ahmad, V. Verma, P. Zeng, S. Ananth, P. Gaur, R. M. Gittelman, E. Yusko, C. Sanders, H. Robins, S. A. Hammond, J. E. Janik, M. Mkrtichyan, S. Gupta, and S. N. Khleif. 2017. Concurrent PD-1 blockade negates the effects of OX40 agonist antibody in combination immunotherapy through inducing T-cell apoptosis. *Cancer Immunology Research* 5(9):755–766.

Shull, J. G. 2019. Digital health and the state of interoperable electronic health records. *JMIR Medical Informatics* 7(4):e12712.

Slaney, C. Y., M. H. Kershaw, and P. K. Darcy. 2014. Trafficking of T cells into tumors. *Cancer Research* 74(24):7168–7174.

Spiegel, J. Y., S. Patel, L. Muffly, M. N. Hossain, J. Oak, J. H. Baird, M. J. Frank, P. Shiraz, B. Sahaf, J. Craig, M. Iglesias, S. Younes, Y. Natkunam, M. G. Ozawa, E. Yang, J. Tamaresis, H. Chinnasamy, Z. Ehlinger, W. Reynolds, R. Lynn, M. C. Rotiroti, N. Gkitsas, S. Arai, L. Johnston, R. Lowsky, R. G. Majzner, E. Meyer, R. S. Negrin, A. R. Rezvani, S. Sidana, J. Shizuru, W. K. Weng, C. Mullins, A. Jacob, I. Kirsch, M. Bazzano, J. Zhou, S. Mackay, S. J. Bornheimer, L. Schultz, S. Ramakrishna, K. L. Davis, K. A. Kong, N. N. Shah, H. Qin, T. Fry, S. Feldman, C. L. Mackall, and D. B. Miklos. 2021. CAR T cells with dual targeting of CD19 and CD22 in adult patients with recurrent or refractory B cell malignancies: A Phase 1 trial. *Nature Medicine* 27(8):1419–1431.

Spiliopoulou, P., S. Y. C. Yang, J. P. Bruce, B. X. Wang, H. K. Berman, T. J. Pugh, and L. L. Siu. 2022. All is not lost: Learning from 9p21 loss in cancer. *Trends in Immunology* 43(5):379–390.

Spreafico, A., A. R. Hansen, A. R. Abdul Razak, P. L. Bedard, and L. L. Siu. 2021. The future of clinical trial design in oncology. *Cancer Discovery* (4):822–837.

Stahlberg, E. A., M. Abdel-Rahman, B. Aguilar, A. Asadpoure, R. A. Beckman, L. L. Borkon, J. N. Bryan, C. M. Cebulla, Y. H. Chang, A. Chatterjee, J. Deng, S. Dolatshahi, O. Gevaert, E. J. Greenspan, W. Hao, T. Hernandez-Boussard, P. R. Jackson, M. Kuijjer, A. Lee, P. Macklin, S. Madhavan, M. D. McCoy, N. Mohammad Mirzaei, T. Razzaghi, H. L. Rocha, L. Shahriari, I. Shmulevich, D. G. Stover, Y. Sun, T. Syeda-Mahmood, J. Wang, Q. Wang, and I. Zervantonakis. 2022. Exploring approaches for predictive cancer patient digital twins: Opportunities for collaboration and innovation. *Frontiers in Digital Health* 4:1007784.

Tarhini, A. A., A. C. Tan, M. Xie, I. El Naqa, P. G. Saghand, D. Dai, J. L. Chen, A. Ratan, M. McCarter, J. D. Carpten, H. Colman, A. Ikeguchi, A. Tripathi, I. Puzanov, S. M. Arnold, M. L. Churchman, P. Hwu, J. Conejo-Garcia, W. S. Dalton, and G. J. Weiner. 2022. Predictors of immunotherapeutic benefits in patients with advanced melanoma and other malignancies treated with immune checkpoint inhibitors utilizing ORIEN "real-world" data. *Journal of Clinical Oncology* 40(16_suppl):2618.

Tawbi, H. A., D. Schadendorf, E. J. Lipson, P. A. Ascierto, L. Matamala, E. Castillo Gutiérrez, P. Rutkowski, H. J. Gogas, C. D. Lao, J. J. De Menezes, S. Dalle, A. Arance, J. J. Grob, S. Srivastava, M. Abaskharoun, M. Hamilton, S. Keidel, K. L. Simonsen, A. M. Sobiesk, B. Li, F. S. Hodi, G. V. Long, and RELATIVITY-047 Investigators. 2022. Relatlimab and nivolumab versus nivolumab in untreated advanced melanoma. *New England Journal of Medicine* 386(1):24–34.

Togashi, Y., K. Shitara, and H. Nishikawa. 2019. Regulatory T cells in cancer immunosuppression—implications for anticancer therapy. *Nature Reviews Clinical Oncology* 16(6):356–371.

Topalian, S. L., J. M. Taube, R. A. Anders, and D. M. Pardoll. 2016. Mechanism-driven biomarkers to guide immune checkpoint blockade in cancer therapy. *Nature Reviews Cancer* 16(5):275–287.

Tsao, M. S., K. M. Kerr, M. Kockx, M. B. Beasley, A. C. Borczuk, J. Botling, L. Bubendorf, L. Chirieac, G. Chen, T. Y. Chou, J. H. Chung, S. Dacic, S. Lantuejoul, M. Mino-Kenudson, A. L. Moreira, A. G. Nicholson, M. Noguchi, G. Pelosi, C. Poleri, P. A. Russell, J. Sauter, E. Thunnissen, I. Wistuba, H. Yu, M. W. Wynes, M. Pintilie, Y. Yatabe, and F. R. Hirsch. 2018. PD-L1 immunohistochemistry comparability study in real-life clinical samples: Results of Blueprint Phase 2 Project. *The Journal of Thoracic Oncology* 13(9):1302–1311.

Upadhaya, S., S. T. Neftelinov, J. Hodge, and J. Campbell. 2022. Challenges and opportunities in the PD1/PDL1 inhibitor clinical trial landscape. *Nature Reviews Drug Discovery* 21(7):482–483.

Vaz, S. C., F. Oliveira, K. Herrmann, and P. Veit-Haibach. 2020. Nuclear medicine and molecular imaging advances in the 21st century. *The British Journal of Radiology* 93(1110):20200095.

Vega, D. M., L. M. Yee, L. M. McShane, P. M. Williams, L. Chen, T. Vilimas, D. Fabrizio, V. Funari, J. Newberg, L. K. Bruce, S. J. Chen, J. Baden, J. C. Barrett, P. Beer, M. Butler, J. H. Cheng, J. Conroy, D. Cyanam, K. Eyring, E. Garcia, G. Green, V. R. Gregersen, M. D. Hellmann, L. A. Keefer, L. Lasiter, A. J. Lazar, M. C. Li, L. E. MacConaill, K. Meier, H. Mellert, S. Pabla, A. Pallavajjala, G. Pestano, R. Salgado, R. Samara, E. S. Sokol, P. Stafford, J. Budczies, A. Stenzinger, W. Tom, K. C. Valkenburg, X. Z. Wang, V. Weigman, M. Xie, Q. Xie, A. Zehir, C. Zhao, Y. Zhao, M. D. Stewart, J. Allen, and TMB Consortium. 2021. Aligning tumor mutational burden (TMB) quantification across diagnostic platforms: Phase II of the Friends of Cancer Research TMB Harmonization Project. *Annals of Oncology* 32(12):1626–1636.

Wang, J., M. F. Sanmamed, I. Datar, T. T. Su, L. Ji, J. Sun, L. Chen, Y. Chen, G. Zhu, W. Yin, L. Zheng, T. Zhou, T. Badri, S. Yao, S. Zhu, A. Boto, M. Sznol, I. Melero, D. A. A. Vignali, K. Schalper, and L. Chen. 2019. Fibrinogen-like protein 1 is a major immune inhibitory ligand of LAG-3. *Cell* 176(1–2):334–347.e12.

Watts, T. H. 2005. TNF/TNFR family members in costimulation of T cell responses. *Annual Review of Immunology* 23:23–68.

Weber, E. W., M. V. Maus, and C. L. Mackall. 2020. The emerging landscape of immune cell therapies. *Cell* 181(1):46–62.

Wei, W., D. Jiang, E. B. Ehlerding, Q. Luo, and W. Cai. 2018. Noninvasive PET imaging of T cells. *Trends in Cancer* 4(5):359–373.

Wei, W., Z. T. Rosenkrans, J. Liu, G. Huang, Q. Y. Luo, and W. Cai. 2020. Immunopet: Concept, design, and applications. *Chemical Reviews* 120(8):3787–3851.

Wherry, E. J. 2011. T cell exhaustion. *Nature Immunology* 12(6):492–499.

William, W. N., Jr., X. Zhao, J. J. Bianchi, H. Y. Lin, P. Cheng, J. J. Lee, H. Carter, L. B. Alexandrov, J. P. Abraham, D. B. Spetzler, S. M. Dubinett, D. W. Cleveland, W. Cavenee, T. Davoli, and S. M. Lippman. 2021. Immune evasion in HPV—head and neck precancer-cancer transition is driven by an aneuploid switch involving chromosome 9p loss. *Proceedings of the National Academy of Sciences* 118(19):e2022655118.

Wolchok, J. D., R. Ibrahim, V. DePril, M. Maio, P. Queirolo, K. Harmankaya, L. Lundgren, A. Hoos, R. Humphrey, and O. Hamid. 2008. Antitumor response and new lesions in advanced melanoma patients on ipilimumab treatment. *Journal of Clinical Oncology* 26(15_suppl):3020.

Wolchok, J. D., A. Hoos, S. O'Day, J. S. Weber, O. Hamid, C. Lebbé, M. Maio, M. Binder, O. Bohnsack, G. Nichol, R. Humphrey, and F. S. Hodi. 2009. Guidelines for the evaluation of immune therapy activity in solid tumors: Immune-related response criteria. *Clinical Cancer Research* 15(23):7412–7420.

Wolchok, J. D., V. Chiarion-Sileni, R. Gonzalez, J. J. Grob, P. Rutkowski, C. D. Lao, C. L. Cowey, D. Schadendorf, J. Wagstaff, R. Dummer, P. F. Ferrucci, M. Smylie, M. O. Butler, A. G. Hill, I. Marquez-Rodas, J. B. A. G. Haanen, T. Bas, W. van Dijck, J. Larkin, and F. S. Hodi. 2021. CheckMate 067: 6.5-year outcomes in patients (pts) with advanced melanoma. *Journal of Clinical Oncology* 39(15_suppl):9506.

Woo, S. R., M. E. Turnis, M. V. Goldberg, J. Bankoti, M. Selby, C. J. Nirschl, M. L. Bettini, D. M. Gravano, P. Vogel, C. L. Liu, S. Tangsombatvisit, J. F. Grosso, G. Netto, M. P. Smeltzer, A. Chaux, P. J. Utz, C. J. Workman, D. M. Pardoll, A. J. Korman, C. G. Drake, and D. A. A. Vignali. 2012. Immune inhibitory molecules LAG-3 and PD-1 synergistically regulate T-cell function to promote tumoral immune escape. *Cancer Research* 72(4):917–927.

Yunna, C., H. Mengru, W. Lei, and C. Weidong. 2020. Macrophage m1/m2 polarization. *European Journal of Pharmacology* 877:173090.

Zappasodi, R., C. Sirard, Y. Li, S. Budhu, M. Abu-Akeel, C. Liu, X. Yang, H. Zhong, W. Newman, J. Qi, P. Wong, D. Schaer, H. Koon, V. Velcheti, M. D. Hellmann, M. A. Postow, M. K. Callahan, J. D. Wolchok, and T. Merghoub. 2019. Rational design of anti-GITR-based combination immunotherapy. *Nature Medicine* 25(5):759–766.

Zhang, Y., R. Kurupati, L. Liu, X. Y. Zhou, G. Zhang, A. Hudaihed, F. Filisio, W. Giles-Davis, X. Xu, G. C. Karakousis, L. M. Schuchter, W. Xu, R. Amaravadi, M. Xiao, N. Sadek, C. Krepler, M. Herlyn, G. J. Freeman, J. D. Rabinowitz, and H. C. J. Ertl. 2017. Enhancing cd8(+) T cell fatty acid catabolism within a metabolically challenging tumor microenvironment increases the efficacy of melanoma immunotherapy. *Cancer Cell* 32(3):377–391.e9.

Zhao, X., E. E. W. Cohen, W. N. William Jr., J. J. Bianchi, J. P. Abraham, D. Magee, D. B. Spetzler, J. S. Gutkind, L. B. Alexandrov, W. K. Cavenee, S. M. Lippman, and T. Davoli. 2022. Somatic 9p24.1 alterations in HPV—head and neck squamous cancer dictate immune microenvironment and anti-PD-1 checkpoint inhibitor activity. *Proceedings of the National Academy of Sciences* 119(47):e2213835119.

Zhou, H., Y. Wang, H. Xu, X. Shen, T. Zhang, X. Zhou, Y. Zeng, K. Li, L. Zhang, H. Zhu, X. Yang, N. Li, Z. Yang, and Z. Liu. 2022. Noninvasive interrogation of CD8+ T cell effector function for monitoring early tumor responses to immunotherapy. *The Journal of Clinical Investigation* 132(16):e161065.

Appendix A

Statement of Task

A National Academies of Sciences, Engineering, and Medicine planning committee will plan and host a 1.5-day public workshop that will examine the current challenges related to resistance to immune modulator therapies for cancer and discuss potential policy levers that could help to overcome these challenges. The workshop will feature invited presentations and panel discussions on topics that may include

- An overview of the unique types of immunotherapy resistance based on the causes of resistance, including whether resistance mechanisms vary among different agents, and gaps in current understanding.
- Policy challenges and opportunities to address the problem of resistance, including
  ○ Criteria to move single agents into clinical trials,
  ○ Criteria to use single agents in combination therapy development (e.g., whether clinical response is necessary),
  ○ Criteria to assess cancer immunotherapy combinations in early-phase clinical trials,
  ○ The roles of preclinical modeling and clinical and predictive biomarkers (e.g., companion diagnostics, in vivo imaging) for assessing safety and efficacy,
  ○ The types of clinical trial designs needed for regulatory approval, and
  ○ Use of big data to aid in determining the dominant drivers of cancer immunotherapy resistance and to predict immunotherapy responses.

The planning committee will develop the agenda for the workshop sessions, select and invite speakers and discussants, and moderate the discussions. A proceedings of the presentations and discussions at the workshop will be prepared by a designated rapporteur in accordance with institutional guidelines.

Appendix B

Workshop Agenda

NOVEMBER 14, 2022

8:30 am   **Welcome from the National Cancer Policy Forum**
Planning Committee Co-Chairs:
- Samir N. Khleif, Georgetown University Medical Center
- George J. Weiner, Holden Comprehensive Cancer Center

8:40 am   **Keynote: Implications of Scientific Innovations on High-Quality Cancer Care and Patient Outcomes**
- Elizabeth M. Jaffee, President's Cancer Panel, Johns Hopkins University (Virtual)

9:00 am   **Session 1: Criteria to Move Single Agents into Clinical Trials**
Co-Moderators:
- Samir N. Khleif, Georgetown University Medical Center
- Tom Curran, Children's Mercy Research Institute, Kansas City University

Single Agent Activity Anti-PD-1
- Suzanne L. Topalian, Johns Hopkins University

Single Agent Activity Anti-Lymphocyte Activation Gene-3 Antibody
- Hussein Tawbi, MD Anderson Cancer Center

Challenges in the Development of Agonist T Cell Antibody Therapy
- John Janik, Cullinan Oncology

Perspective on Resistance to CAR T: Lessons from Blood Cancer
- Stephan A. Grupp, Children's Hospital of Philadelphia (Virtual)

FDA Regulatory Perspective: What Has Changed and What Is Missing?
- Peter F. Bross, Center for Biologics Evaluation and Research, Food and Drug Administration

Panel Discussion

10:30 am   **Break**

10:40 am   **Session 2: Current Challenges and Opportunities: Selection of Experimental Agents in Combinations**
Co-Moderators:
- Gideon Blumenthal, Merck
- Marc Theoret, Oncology Center of Excellence, Food and Drug Administration

Understanding Immune Therapy Efficacy, Preclinical Models, and Combination Resistance
- Samir N. Khleif, Georgetown University Medical Center

Clinical Trials in PD-1/L1 Refractory Cancers
- Jane A. Healy, Merck Research Labs

Anti-PD-1 and Epacadostat vs. IDO Inhibition: Lessons Learned
- Jason J. Luke, University of Pittsburgh Medical Center

Intralesional Approaches: Regulatory Issues
- George J. Weiner, Holden Comprehensive Cancer Center

Panel Discussion

12:00 pm   **Break**

1:00 pm	**Session 3: Current Challenges and Opportunities: Biomarkers and Surrogate Endpoints**

Co-Moderators:
- Kimryn Rathmell, Vanderbilt University Medical Center
- Chris Boshoff, Pfizer Inc (Virtual)

Genetic Biomarkers: 9p21 Loss Drives Immune-Cold, Checkpoint-Inhibitor Resistance in HPV Head and Neck Squamous Cancer
- Teresa Davoli, NYU Langone Health (Virtual)

Diagnostic Imaging
- Marius Mayerhoefer, Memorial Sloan Kettering Cancer Center

Immune Metabolism
- Hildegund C.J. Ertl, The Wistar Institute

Novel Surrogate Biomarkers for Immune Therapy Response and Resistance
- Kimryn Rathmell, Vanderbilt University Medical Center

Biomarkers and Imaging: Current Regulatory Landscape
- Reena Philip, Oncology Center of Excellence, Food and Drug Administration

Surrogate Endpoint Development
- Nicole Gormley, Oncology Center of Excellence, Food and Drug Administration

Panel Discussion

2:40 pm	**Break**

2:50 pm	**Session 4: Current Challenges and Opportunities: The Role of Data and Computational Tools**

Co-Moderators:
- Nancy E. Davidson, Fred Hutchinson Cancer Center
- Julie R. Gralow, American Society of Clinical Oncology

Regulatory and Access Considerations in Mining Big Data
- Ahmad A. Tarhini, H. Lee Moffitt Cancer Center and Research Institute

Advanced Computing Tools
- Jack D. Hidary, SandboxAQ (Virtual)

Data-Driven Approaches for Modeling Response and Resistance
- Dana Pe'er, Memorial Sloan Kettering Cancer Center

Leveraging Real-World Data to Characterize Immune Related Adverse Events
- Prakirthi Yerram, Flatiron Health

AI, Data Science, and Big Data Approaches to Accelerate and Expand Research and Evaluation
- Usama Fayyad, Institute for Experiential Artificial Intelligence at Northeastern University

Panel Discussion

4:20 pm   **Closing Remarks**
Planning Committee Co-Chairs:
- Samir N. Khleif, Georgetown University Medical Center
- George J. Weiner, Holden Comprehensive Cancer Center

4:30 pm   **Adjourn**

NOVEMBER 15, 2022

8:30 am   **Welcome and Overview of Day 2**
Planning Committee Co-Chairs:
- Samir N. Khleif, Georgetown University Medical Center
- George J. Weiner, Holden Comprehensive Cancer Center

8:40 am   **Session 5: Criteria to Assess Cancer Immunotherapy Combinations in Early-Phase Clinical Trial Designs Needed for Regulatory Approval**
Co-Moderators:
- Roy S. Herbst, Yale Comprehensive Cancer Center (Virtual)
- Hedvig Hricak, Memorial Sloan Kettering Cancer Center

Novel Immunotherapy Clinical Trial Design
- Keith T. Flaherty, Massachusetts General Hospital; Harvard Medical School

Public–Private Partnership Perspective
- Roy Herbst, Yale Comprehensive Cancer Center (Virtual)

Selected Regulatory Considerations for Cancer Immunotherapeutic Combinations: Contribution of Individual Components to Effect of Combination
- Marc Theoret, Oncology Center of Excellence, Food and Drug Administration

National Cancer Institute Perspective on Novel Trial Designs for Immunotherapy Resistance
- Elad Sharon, NCI Cancer Therapy Evaluation Program

An Industry Perspective
- Alexandra Snyder, Generate Biomedicines

Challenges of Trial Design: Incorporating Pharmacodynamics
- Jedd Wolchok, Weill Cornell Medicine (Virtual)

Panel Discussion

10:10 am **Break**

10:20 am **Session 6: Panel Discussion**
Reflections on the Workshop and Next Steps to Overcome Resistance to Immune Modulator Therapies for Cancer Treatment
Co-Moderators:
- George J. Weiner, Holden Comprehensive Cancer Center
- Scott M. Lippman, University of California, San Diego

Panelists:
- Session 1: Samir N. Khleif and Tom Curran
- Session 2: Gideon Blumenthal and Marc Theoret
- Session 3: Kimryn Rathmell and Chris Boshoff (Virtual)
- Session 4: Nancy E. Davidson and Julie R. Gralow
- Session 5: Roy S. Herbst (Virtual) and Hedvig Hricak

Open Discussion

11:50 am   **Closing Remarks**
Planning Committee Co-Chairs:
- Samir N. Khleif, Georgetown University Medical Center
- George J. Weiner, Holden Comprehensive Cancer Center

12:00 pm   **Adjourn**